Alison Roberts has been lucky enough to live in the South of France for several years recently, but is now back in her home country of New Zealand. She is also lucky enough to write for the Mills & Boon Medical line. A primary school teacher in a former life, she later became a qualified paramedic. She loves to travel and dance, drink champagne and spend time with her daughter and her friends. Alison is the author of over one hundred books!

Also by Alison Roberts

Therapy Pup to Heal the Surgeon
City Vet, Country Temptation
Paramedic's Reunion in Paradise
Midwife's Three-Date Rule
Their Fake Date Rescue

A Tale of Two Midwives miniseries

Falling for Her Forbidden Flatmate
Miracle Twins to Heal Them

Royal York Hospital collection

Single Dad's Christmas Wish

Discover more at millsandboon.co.uk.

A FAMILY MADE IN THE ER

ALISON ROBERTS

SINGLE DAD FOR THE DAREDEVIL DOCTOR

ALISON ROBERTS

MILLS & BOON

First published in Great Britain 2026
by Mills & Boon, an imprint of HarperCollins*Publishers* Ltd,
1 London Bridge Street, London, SE1 9GF

www.harpercollins.co.uk

HarperCollins*Publishers* Macken House, 39/40 Mayor Street Upper,
Dublin 1, D01 C9W8, Ireland

A Family Made in the ER © 2026 Alison Roberts

Single Dad for the Daredevil Doctor © 2026 Alison Roberts

ISBN: 978-0-263-41979-5

01/26

This book contains FSC™ certified paper
and other controlled sources to ensure responsible forest management.

For more information visit www.harpercollins.co.uk/green.

Printed and Bound in the UK using 100% Renewable Electricity
at CPI Group (UK) Ltd, Croydon, CR0 4YY

A FAMILY
MADE IN THE ER

ALISON ROBERTS

MILLS & BOON

CHAPTER ONE

THE PATIENT WAS *in severe respiratory distress.*

He was sitting upright on the ambulance stretcher, leaning forward. Gasping as he held a mask to his face, his features blurred by the mist of nebulised medication he was trying to inhale.

'Thirty-nine-year-old male.' The tone of the lead paramedic's voice as he started his verbal transfer indicated how urgent this case was. 'Asthmatic but it's usually controlled by inhalers. Sudden onset of symptoms. Heart rate one forty, resp rate thirty-six, blood pressure one sixty on eighty-five. Oxygen saturation falling, currently on ninety-two percent.'

Alex took command of the situation in his usual confident style.

'Resus One,' he directed the crew. 'Riley, activate a Code Blue, please.'

Riley went into the resuscitation area herself seconds later, having put out the urgent alarm to summon the rest of the team on call for a critical medical event. The patient had already been transferred to the bed. Alex was getting more information from the paramedics.

'No other medical history of note. He smokes ten cigarettes a day.'

Riley sneaked a peek at Alex's face. She knew, better than anyone else in this room, what he thought of people who were stupid enough to keep smoking when they had a chronic respiratory disease like asthma but there was no sign of judgement on his face. Of course there wasn't. His consummate professionalism and skill in what was such a demanding profession was one of the things that had attracted her to him in the first place.

'Is that IV line patent?'

'Not now. He was agitated enough to try pulling it out.'

'We need another one. Stat. And an arterial line. Get me—'

'Heart rate's dropping,' a voice called. 'Increasing ectopics.'

Riley's breath caught in her throat as her gaze swerved towards the overhead monitor. Yes...the trace of the heart rhythm on the screen was being disrupted at frequent intervals by the bizarrely shaped squiggles of abnormal beats. The patient's level of consciousness was dropping and his chin was slowly dipping as if his head was now too heavy to hold up.

'Silent chest.' Alex removed the earpieces of his stethoscope with a flick of one hand. 'He's not moving any air.' He lifted his gaze to look directly at Riley.

She gave a single nod. She knew she had to prepare for the imminent possibility of a cardiopulmonary arrest. They would need to start CPR, intubate their patient, start an aggressive protocol of medication and—

* * *

What *was* that insistent noise? Oh, of course…it was the vibration of a hard object against the wooden top of her desk.

With a sound that was very close to a frustrated growl, Isla Preston's fingers stilled on her keyboard and reached for the phone.

She'd put it on silent but hadn't thought to kill the vibration mode. Now completely distracted, she picked up the device with a sigh of defeat. This was the first time in nearly a week that she'd had a chance to get some work done on her latest book and the words were just beginning to flow. They *needed* to flow. Isla never missed a deadline and this one was getting inexorably closer with every passing week.

But she couldn't ignore her phone even if she wasn't rostered on any level of call. Not when she was one of the senior doctors in a currently understaffed emergency department in a small regional hospital. What if there was some kind of major incident happening like a bus crash or building collapse? She couldn't ignore this any more than she'd been able to refuse to take on too many extra shifts when the HoD of Coromandel Hospital's ED had been suddenly called back to the UK in response to a family emergency.

She stared at the caller ID on her screen to find it was none other than the HoD himself, Jake Hammond.

'Hallelujah,' Isla muttered. Maybe Jake was back from the UK already and she'd be able to return to her part-time position in the emergency department, pull up the drawbridge and sink into the solitude and peace of her side hustle of writing medical thrillers.

Isla swiped the screen. 'Jake? Hey…where are you?' She couldn't help a hopeful tone. 'Are you back in New Zealand already?'

'Hi, Isla. No, I'm still in Bristol.'

'Oh…' Her heart sank. And then she gave herself a mental slap for being so selfish. 'Sorry to hear that. Are you okay?'

It felt a little odd to be asking such a personal question. Jake had started work in the Thames Coromandel district hospital nearly a year ago now but it wasn't that often they worked together because they were the two most senior consultants so she usually covered his days off. They were friendly enough but not exactly *friends*. Because Isla didn't have friends. The professional environment of working with colleagues and patients when she was on shift was quite enough human contact for her. Out of work hours she preferred to be alone.

Tucked away in her personal haven. Immersed in the worlds she created for the characters in her books.

'Not exactly…' Jake sounded tired. Or down? 'I'm actually ringing to warn you that I'll be away for longer than I thought.'

Isla closed her eyes and didn't say anything for a moment. A moment that was probably long enough to make her disappointment quite obvious. Long enough for Jake to step in to fill the silence, anyway.

'I know… I had no idea what I was going to find when I got here.' She could hear Jake's heavy sigh. 'And now things have taken a bit of a turn for the worse. My brother died last night.'

'Oh, my God… I'm *so* sorry.' She'd known that his brother and his family had been involved in a nasty car accident. She'd heard that his sister-in-law had died at the scene and his brother was in the intensive care unit, listed as being in a critical condition. And wasn't there a child involved as well?

'There's all the funeral arrangements to sort,' Jake said. 'And that takes time over here, but what's worse is that my nephew isn't doing so well. Arlo. He's only nine, poor kid, and he's lost both his parents.'

Isla could feel herself stiffening. She didn't want to hear about his nine-year-old nephew. She almost wanted to put her fingers in her ears and go 'la, la, la…' How immature was *that*?

She couldn't tune out Jake's voice, however much she might want to.

'So it turns out he was born with only one kidney. No one knew until he had a CT scan to find out where his abdominal bleeding was coming from, which was his spleen and his liver. That got dealt with in Theatre but now his kidney's failing. He's probably going to need to go onto dialysis. I'm going to get myself tested tomorrow to see if I'm a potential donor if things deteriorate further but, even if I am, it's not something that could happen until he's through this crisis.' The sigh was even more heartfelt this time. 'Anyway…it's not your problem. I just want to know how you're coping. It could be a month before I can get back. I can ask for management to find a locum. Or I could resign and let them offer a permanent position, but that might take a lot longer.'

'No…don't resign. Please…' It had been hard enough to find someone who wanted to live and work this far away from a major city, let alone someone who was as good at his job as Jake was. 'I'm coping. And Sam's cancelled her holidays to cover you until you get back. *We're* coping.'

It was true.

Okay, she'd never planned to work full-time again and she might not be getting enough time to work on her book but that wasn't really the end of the world, was it? She could ask her editor for an extension to her deadline and the extra cash from working more hours would come in handy to finally do the roof replacement on her house that had been flagged as urgent a year ago.

'Are you sure?' For the first time in this conversation, Isla could hear a more positive note in Jake's voice and it made her feel better too. He was having a far worse time than she would be for the next few weeks. She knew, too well, how hard it could be to navigate grief and jump through all the personal and bureaucratic hoops to try and keep putting one foot in front of the other. Not that Jake was aware, but this gave them a bond that, however unwelcome it might be, she was powerless to prevent wrapping itself around her heart.

'I'm sure,' she said quietly. 'Don't worry about anything here, Jake, and…take care of yourself, okay? I hope things come right for your nephew very soon.'

'So do I.' Jake's words were heartfelt. 'He's the only family I've got left.'

It was the crack in his voice that was too much for Isla. 'Best of luck,' she said quickly. 'Call me if there's anything I can do to help, other than cover your shifts, like...' She was thinking fast, wanting to end this call. 'Like watering any plants you've got at your place?'

A huff of something like laughter came from Jake. 'Don't do pot plants,' he said. 'Or pets. I've managed to avoid any kind of dependents for my entire adult life. How ironic is that?'

And now he was the only family for a child? It *was* ironic. The information was also far too personal for Isla to be comfortable responding to.

'Okay... Sorry, Jake, but I've got to go. I've got someone at the door. Take care...'

She ended the call and then sat for a long, long moment, her head bowed. Someone at the door?

As if.

It was precisely why she lived in this isolated little house above a beach, an hour's drive away from work. On a good day, that was. The road was prone to slips in bad weather and winding enough to collect an above average score of serious car accidents, but fortunately scenarios like that didn't happen often. Allowing extra time for travel was usually enough to let her manage and it was worth any hassles.

Nobody was going to intrude on her privacy here. Most people didn't even know there was a house tucked into the edge of a native forest, which was why her grandparents had built it as a weekend retreat to escape the rat race in Auckland. She'd spent every holiday of her childhood here and it had been her permanent home for five years now. An escape that had been a lifesaver.

A few more deep breaths and Isla lifted her head again. She stared at the words on the computer screen in front of her and then began rereading what she'd been writing before the phone call had interrupted her. It should be easy enough to get back into the scene. She had a full-on medical drama to write and, somewhere in that controlled chaos, Doctor Alex was about to murder a patient in full view of an entire resus team, including the woman he was in an intimate relationship with. And Riley would have no idea that their patient had died of anything other than an acute asthma attack that had simply been too difficult to reverse.

Isla put her fingers back on the keyboard and started typing.

The sooner she could immerse herself in this fantasy world again, the happier she would be.

Jake Hammond was no stranger to the subdued atmosphere of an intensive care unit where there was a fight for life going on in almost every bedspace. He'd loved the drama of those fights as a doctor and had spent years as a consultant in one of the busiest ICUs in New Zealand after heading to the other side of the world for a new life.

It had been a shock, mind you, to be beside one of these beds surrounded by state-of-the-art monitoring systems as a relative and not in a professional capacity. Not just one bed either. Ever since he'd arrived from over thirty hours of non-stop travelling, he'd shuttled from one glass cubicle to another.

One bed held his nephew, Arlo. His younger brother, Troy, had been in the other. Ironically, Troy had decided Jake was a complete failure as a brother when he'd been about Arlo's age. How much had he told his son about his own childhood? Enough that he'd be the last person Arlo would want to be caring for him when he woke up?

If he woke up...?

Jake closed his eyes, his head bowed, as he rubbed his forehead with his fingers, but then he lifted his chin and opened his eyes. His gaze was steady as he looked at the mop of black hair, long enough to be fanned out on the white pillow. Arlo's eyelashes were black, too, resting on cheeks that were almost as pale as the pillow.

'I did do my best for your dad.' His voice was no more than a whisper. 'But I'll do better for you, if you'll let me.'

Or if anyone else would let him. Arlo might be the only family Jake had left in the world but Social Services were still trying to find any contacts on his mother's side. Maybe a grandparent or other close relative was going to appear any day now and claim guardianship rights.

Would that be a relief?

Jake was honest enough to admit that it probably would be, but there was another line of thought that was becoming stronger as the hours were ticking past and he listened to the soft sound of Arlo's heartbeat coming from one of the bank of monitors around him and the hiss and click of the ventilator that was breathing for him.

He might have failed his younger brother, and he could never erase that from his life story, but this was beginning to feel as if it could be a chance to at least go some way to making up for that. He'd been no more than a child himself back then, when it had all fallen apart. He was a lot older now. Hopefully a lot wiser.

Arlo looked so like Troy had at this age. How old had his kid brother been when they'd been separated to go into different foster homes? Jake had been fourteen, so Troy would have been eight. A year younger than Arlo was now. So young.

So heartbreakingly vulnerable.

Jake wasn't going to fail this time. He was going to take this second chance and not let history repeat itself.

The snake's nest of tubes and wires connecting Arlo to the monitors didn't bother Jake because he understood the purpose of each of them. The expression on the consultant's face as he came quietly into the room did bother him—because he understood that, too.

He took the laboratory result form that was being offered and blew out a breath when he saw the results of the kidney function tests.

'We're going to start CRRT,' the consultant said. 'The nephrology team is on its way.'

Jake nodded. Continuous Renal Replacement Therapy was more gentle on the body than filtering the blood by other forms of dialysis and it was becoming the gold standard for kidney failure in paediatric critical care.

'We'll insert a femoral cannula. Hopefully, it'll only be for a few days until Arlo's kidney starts functioning again. If it's needed long-term, we can start talking about a transplant.' The consultant raised an eyebrow. 'You've had bloods taken for the first stage of donor matching?'

'Yes.' Jake's nod was curt. 'Blood group compatibility is confirmed. I'm waiting for the results of the first serum cross-match test. If Arlo's serum reacts with my white blood cells, then I'll be crossed off the list of potential donors, but I'm hoping some other close relatives on his mother's side are being tracked down in case that happens.' His smile was wry. 'I thought I knew how hard this kind of thing was on families.' He shook his head. 'I had no idea.'

'It's a steep learning curve all right, being on the other side of the equation. Ahh...' The consultant looked up as a new machine was wheeled into the room. A big gun in the arsenal of weapons to try and keep Arlo alive. Empty bags were attached that would soon be full of blood as it was taken from Arlo's body and then returned, with waste products like urea and creatinine removed, via more tubes. There was more medication to get pumped into that small body as well, including an anticoagulant to stop any clots forming in his blood.

The room was now crowded with doctors and technicians.

Someone gave Jake a sympathetic smile. 'You don't have to stay if you'd rather not,' they said. 'It's a bit of an invasive procedure, getting this set up.'

Jake could still hear the quiet word someone else had with the speaker. 'He's a doctor, not just the kid's uncle. ICU and emergency expert.'

Nobody suggested he left after that, but Jake went to the head of the bed so he wasn't going to get in anyone's way.

He watched them setting up and prepping that delicate skin on Arlo's groin that would be cut to insert the large dual-lumen catheter. Distracting himself by thinking about what was going to happen tomorrow was helpful. He had a meeting with the people from Social Services in the morning. And a funeral director. A counsellor had offered an appointment. So had the hospital chaplain. People were surrounding him with support so why did he feel so incredibly alone?

As if it was just him and Arlo against the world?

CHAPTER TWO

IT WAS NOT uncommon for tropical cyclones to form north of New Zealand but these destructive storms usually weakened significantly before they made landfall on the eastern coastline of the North Island. Any concern that they might be in for some severe weather, however, resulted in all emergency services and hospitals being notified and one such notification had arrived for Coromandel Hospital earlier this week. The wind and rain had been increasing steadily over the last couple of days.

'Maybe I should stay here overnight, Sam,' Isla suggested. 'There's always a spare bed in the staff quarters.'

But Sam shook her head. 'Forecast at the moment is that it's changing direction and it shouldn't get much worse than this, but if any road is likely to get cut off in a storm it's the stretch between here and your side of the peninsula, and if that happens your expertise in emergency medicine would be a vital resource for the whole of the east coast.'

Samantha Gillespie, their new senior emergency department registrar, was speaking with the authority that came with her position in LandSAR—the specialist volunteer search and rescue organisation that could be activated and coordinated by the national police and rescue services in any emergency involving people that were lost, missing or injured. She'd been involved with the organisation for years in Auckland and the local members had welcomed her on board.

Isla bit her lip, pretending to be scanning the whiteboard as if the number of patients they had under their care and what treatment they were receiving might be the deciding factor of where her skills were really needed. She was, however, really pushing down a flutter of something like panic. The very last thing she wanted to get caught up in was a rescue scenario on the coast—or worse, at sea. Five years had not been anywhere near long enough for the nightmare of her personal brush with death to fade. Flashbacks were far less frequent, of course, but they hadn't lost any of their gut-wrenching punch.

'Is your kit fully stocked?'

'Yes.' Isla's solid four-wheel-drive utility vehicle with a locked canopy over its deck was almost as well stocked as an ambulance as far as the range of first response equipment and drugs went. 'I just replaced the oxygen cylinder today,' she added.

'Good.' Sam's nod was brisk. 'I'll get you a satellite phone for backup communication.'

She must have seen the indecision on Isla's face. 'Hey…don't worry about us. I'm going to admit that guy with the chest infection and exacerbation of COPD and discharge our friend who's slept off the effects of his overindulgence at the pub last night. We can get extra help down from Auckland if we need it for a natural disaster and if the roads are closed and the weather gets too bad to fly, there are a lot of communities on your side of the peninsula that will be relying on a very small pool of medics.'

Isla nodded. It was true. Sam was more than capable of being left in charge of the emergency department here. In her thirties, like Isla, Sam had started out as a general practitioner in Auckland before deciding to follow her passion and do postgraduate training in emergency medicine. She was skilled, ambitious and devoted to her career. She was also a very nice person. If Isla was going to let someone close enough to share her life as a friend, then Sam would be at the top of the list but, so far, it had been easy to swerve the temptation.

Sam probably wouldn't be around for long enough, anyway. She hadn't made any secret of the fact that being in a regional hospital was merely a stepping stone for her to get back to the bright lights and guaranteed drama a big city could provide. Isla could see that she was, on some level, relishing the prospect of a weather-related challenge ahead. Maybe she was secretly hoping the weather forecast was wrong in predicting the storm might change course in the next few hours and head further out to sea.

'And hey…' Sam pulled out an ace from her sleeve. 'Jake's on his way back. He might have landed in Auckland already.'

'I didn't know that.' The wash of relief was surprisingly strong. 'What happened about his nephew? It's been weeks since I spoke to him.'

'I haven't caught up on that. I just heard that he rang Polly in Admin yesterday and said he'd be back on board this week. He might even drop in tomorrow. If he's in town and he's needed, we both know nothing will stop him being here.'

'Okay…' That made all the difference. 'In that case, I will head over the hills.'

'Great. Let me get you that phone. I'll find some overalls and boots for you, too. Just in case…' She shook her head. 'I hope Jake hasn't ended up with a kid to look after. That would be my worst nightmare ever.'

'Yeah…' It was probably a good thing that Isla had already turned away and Sam couldn't see her face. 'Mine, too.'

'Are we there yet?'

'Nearly.'

Jake slowed his car as they reached yet another uphill hairpin bend. There were only two roads that went across the peninsula to join the coastal roads and they were both a bit hairy. This one went through the Coromandel Forest Park, which was spectacular but slow going. They'd still get to their destination well before dark, however, and hopefully before this storm got any worse. It was still raining hard enough to need the wipers on their fastest speed. The other slight issues that Jake hadn't put too much time into thinking about yet were that fishing the address for Dr Isla Preston out of the internal hospital computer system had not only been breaking a rule or two but it also looked as if the property might be rather difficult to locate.

Was it totally off the grid? The upside-down teardrop pin on the satellite map seemed to be in the middle of a swathe of native bush with its only access looking more like a walking track than a road, or possibly just a beach. Maybe he should have waited until he could have seen her at work. A private office at the hospital would have worked just as well for what he needed to talk to her about, wouldn't it?

No. He'd already had this conversation with himself. More than once.

He had the feeling that what he had to tell Isla Preston would be as much of a shock to her as it had been to him and he had absolutely no idea how she was going to react. It had made him realise how little he really knew about a colleague he'd worked with for more than a year now, and that made him wonder whether part of that was his fault. Had he become too good at keeping professional boundaries in place? Had he made even more of an effort as far as Isla Preston was concerned because she was an attractive single woman and having anything more than a purely professional relationship with someone he worked with was not something that could be easily brushed aside in such a small town?

Whatever. It was only good manners to let anyone absorb what could be life-changing information in a private space. Part of the human decency that had made Jake decide this also had to be a face-to-face meeting rather than anything handled in written form, either by himself or, even worse, by a legal firm.

Emerging from the forest, the land began to flatten out and it was possible to go faster. There might be a few one-lane bridges to get across numerous rivers but it wouldn't take long to get to the township of Tairua.

Not that Isla lived anywhere near its periphery. No… he had to go through the town, head for the autumnal-sounding area called Pumpkin Hill and then take a road that wound its way through another forest. He got Arlo to watch the sat nav for him as they left the beachside town behind.

'There might be a road sign for Te Karo Bay or it might say Sailors Grave Beach,' he said. 'That's where we're heading.'

'Why's it called Sailors Grave Beach?'

'I guess a sailor got buried there.'

Arlo's grunt was unimpressed. No surprises there. Arlo had been unimpressed with everything Jake had done in the last few weeks, ever since he'd regained consciousness to find that an uncle he had no memory of ever meeting was now his only relative. And that, when he was well enough, he was going to be taken away from his home and school and friends—his entire world, in fact—to live on what might as well be a different planet. He was, understandably, a very confused and frightened young boy.

'*Putting you into foster care isn't an option,*' Jake had explained as gently as he could. '*You might not remember me but I am your family. You might have other family but probably not here in the UK, seeing as your mum came from New Zealand. If it turns out that you hate it there, we can talk about moving back here but I can't just walk out on my job any more than I can walk out on you. Sorry, buddy, but you don't have a choice. Especially when you're still recovering from being so sick.*'

Physically, he'd recovered surprisingly fast once he'd

turned the corner after a couple of days of dialysis. Losing his parents had been an emotional blow the poor kid was nowhere near coming to terms with, and he was still too quiet and withdrawn, but Jake knew that it would take time. The fact that Arlo hadn't shut himself away completely or gone completely off the rails and refused to cooperate at all spoke volumes about his courage and character, along with a commendable maturity for a nine-year-old.

Not that Arlo would want to hear it, any more than he'd allow himself to be hugged, but Jake was proud of him. He was totally committed to keeping his nephew safe and being there for him for as long as he was needed. He was also determined to track down any other relatives that Arlo might have. The news that he was not suitable to donate a kidney if it was needed in the future had been disappointing enough to make him put more effort into a search that had taken a very unexpected twist just the day before they were due to get on their long-haul flight to the small country at the bottom of the world. It was either a red herring or the kind of ridiculous coincidence that could only happen in fiction rather than real life but it was on the top of his list of things that needed sorting—preferably before he was back at work in the next few days.

'We're nearly at the turnoff,' Arlo muttered.

'Thanks. I see it.' The branches on the trees that lined the road as they headed downhill again were being pummelled by wind gusts. They couldn't see the beach as they reached the bay but they could hear the roar of angry surf as they went past a parking area and a small building that looked as if it could be a public toilet. The road narrowed after that and there was no sign of habitation.

'Keep an eye out for a driveway.' Jake was driving as slowly as he could, peering through the heavy sheets of water being sloshed off the windscreen. 'I don't think there'll be a letterbox, but you never know. It's the last house before the road ends so I don't think we can miss it.'

They couldn't. It had a signpost. 'Private Property' was painted in white lettering on a plank of wood nailed to a tree trunk. It didn't say that trespassers would be prosecuted and it didn't have a skull and crossbones to warn them to stay out but Jake found himself taking a deep breath before he turned and drove off the road.

When he stopped the car, he turned to Arlo. 'Stay in the car for a minute or two, okay?'

'Why?'

'I need to see if the person who lives here is home.'

'You mean you don't know?'

'No.'

'So we might have driven all this way for nothing? That's nuts.'

'Maybe. Maybe not.'

Jake opened his car door, preparing to make a dash to the door. He had a horrible feeling that Arlo might be right. This *was* nuts.

There was nothing better than the sound of rain on a corrugated iron roof. It was one of Isla Preston's favourite things in life, in fact.

Especially when the log burner was stoked and the whole house felt warm. She had her laptop and mobile phone fully charged in case the power went out later. The local medical centre had her number and she had the satellite phone if she was needed to join any search and rescue mission but, with a bit of luck, there would be no sting in the tail of this particular cyclone and this wild weather would have blown itself out by morning.

She might have an entire evening to work on her book. Having mapped a lot of it out now, Isla was going back to refine a few of the clues she was scattering into the plot. Like the random glass ampoule her heroine, Riley, had found on the floor of the resuscitation area in the sombre aftermath of an unexpected fatality in a young and otherwise fit man.

'Where on earth did this come from?'

'Probably just got dropped. Hardly unusual in a full-on cardiac arrest situation. We both know what that's like.'

'But this is for a beta blocker.' Riley couldn't ignore the faint alarm bell sounding in the back of her mind. Any doctor knew that beta-blockers were drugs that could create or exacerbate an asthma attack. They certainly had no place in either a treatment protocol for asthma or dealing with a cardiac and respiratory arrest.

'Must have been missed cleaning up after an earlier case. Heart failure, maybe. Or a hypertensive crisis?'

'Yeah... I guess so. Must have been before I came on duty, though.' Riley should have put the small glass

ampoule with its snapped-off neck into the sharps container on the bench but, for some reason, she slipped it into her pocket. Should she ask Alex about it? No... he'd been the lead doctor in a case that had ended in tragedy. She knew him well enough by now to know that talking about it was a no-go area at home. She also knew he was oversensitive to anything he perceived to be personal criticism.

When had it started feeling as if she was walking on eggshells sometimes?

Isla reached for her coffee cup to take a sip. The latest squall seemed to have passed and the rattle of rain on the roof was fading. Enough for her to hear the knock on her door, anyway.

She froze for an instant. Nobody came knocking on her door. Very few people knew where she lived. It wasn't likely that anyone was at the beach today, or using the walking track that joined onto her road and had come looking for help. Was it one of the few neighbours she had along this isolated road?

Cautiously, Isla opened her door a little, ready to slam it shut if it was a stranger and her instincts were sounding a warning.

It wasn't a stranger.

But her alarm bells were going off just like her heroine Riley's had been a minute or two ago.

'*Jake?* What the hell...?'

'Sorry to turn up out of blue like this, Isla.'

She knew her expression had to be incredulous, and

it wasn't because he'd driven this far in less than ideal weather conditions.

'How did you find out where I live?'

He looked guilty. Had he got unauthorised access to her personal information? If so, it was totally unacceptable and she would be making a formal complaint.

'One question,' he said. 'If the answer's no I'll apologise for intruding and make myself scarce. If it's yes you might prefer that we have a private conversation.'

What on earth was he on about? Isla didn't open the door any further but she didn't slam it shut either. She simply stared at Jake.

'Have you got a sister?' he asked. 'Called Sage? Sage McGregor?'

Isla's jaw dropped. It took her a moment to realise how dim-witted she must look, standing there staring at Jake with her mouth hanging open. She closed it, pressed her lips together tightly and swallowed. Hard.

'Yes.' Her voice was only a whisper. 'But I lost touch with her. Years ago.'

'Is this her?'

Jake had a passport in his hand. A New Zealand passport. He opened it to the photo page and Isla covered her mouth with her hand to stifle her gasp. How could Jake possibly have known about the relationship? And why was *he* here—with her sister's passport? She pulled the door open further. 'Um…maybe you'd better come inside.'

Jake looked over his shoulder. 'I…ah… I've got someone in the car…'

Isla could actually feel the blood draining from her

face now. 'Sage?' she asked. 'Have you got my *sister* in your car?'

'Oh, God…no…' Jake's face creased into distressed lines. 'I'm so sorry, Isla. I'm making a right mess of this. I came all the way here because I have news I didn't think you'd want to hear in a more public place. Bad news, I'm afraid.'

Isla was holding onto the door to steady herself. 'About Sage?'

'Yes. I'm sorry.' He gestured at the old armchair on the veranda. 'Do you want to sit down?'

She ignored the invitation. 'What's happened to Sage?'

'She was in a car accident. She was killed instantly. They couldn't trace any relatives and your name only came up a couple of days ago after a lead on social media. I wasn't even sure it was you—there are any number of people out there with the same name—but, if it was, I didn't want you to get the news from a couple of police officers turning up at the hospital.'

Isla managed a nod. She didn't know how to start processing this news. Or how she felt, even. Sad, of course…but it was over ten years since she'd had any contact with Sage and guilt was currently overriding grief. She should have tried harder to find her little sister. She *had* been trying…until her own life had been so utterly derailed.

'There's something else you need to know, too.' Jake was watching her carefully. There was empathy in his gaze. And concern. Was he trying to gauge whether she could handle another shock?

Of course she could. Isla felt numb. She'd dealt with worse than this. The grief would come later, when she was on her own, and she knew she would cope with that as well. She had enough experience, hadn't she?

'What?' The question was more like a demand.

'The person I have in my car is Sage's son. Your nephew.'

Isla was staring at Jake again. Without blinking. She saw a flash of something in Jake's eyes but, for the life of her, she couldn't interpret the emotion.

'He's my nephew too,' Jake said. 'His father was my brother. Sage's partner.'

She couldn't say a word. He'd told her what his nephew's name was, hadn't he?

Arlo...

It had occurred to her at the time that it was probably the closest male equivalent to her own name. Maybe now, she knew why. Had Sage named her son after her sister? No. She didn't want to even think about that. About a connection to this child that she really, really didn't want. She could feel her face scrunching with her determination to ignore the thought.

The flash of lightning, closely followed by the rumble of thunder, was like a plot device Isla might have put into one of her stories for dramatic effect. It made this whole scenario feel like fiction rather than real life, but she couldn't push a delete button and make this disappear, could she?

'I suppose you'd better bring him inside too, then,' she said.

CHAPTER THREE

'*Wait!*'

Jake had only got back to his vehicle to tell Arlo he could come inside now when he heard the door of the house slam behind him. He turned to see Isla pulling on a heavy rainproof jacket. He recognised the distinctive aerial of a satellite phone on the device she was holding.

'I've got to go,' she said. 'I've had a call from our local police. They're at the scene of a car versus motorbike and the ambulance crew's requested assistance. Air rescue's at least thirty minutes away and the local GP's waiting for a patient with unstable angina and chest pain to arrive at the medical centre.'

She pointed her remote key at the big black ute that Jake had parked behind and its hazard lights flashed as it beeped and unlocked itself.

Jake's response was automatic. 'I'll come with you.'

'You don't want to get caught up at an accident scene when you've got your nephew to look after.'

His nephew? Had she just dismissed her own relationship to Arlo? Jake could feel his eyes narrowing. Maybe his sympathy at having to deliver bad news to Isla had been misplaced. She had exactly the same link and therefore responsibility towards this child as he did.

How dare she just dismiss it? He opened his mouth to say something but Isla beat him to it.

'If you could shift your car, I'll be able to get out,' Isla said, pulling open her driver's door. 'We can talk later. Tomorrow, maybe? At work?'

Jake didn't get a chance to say anything before Isla got into her vehicle and slammed the door shut. He got into his car and backed off to give her room to turn around. She paused for a moment to reach out of her window and place a large magnetic light on the roof. It was flashing red a second later and she was heading down her driveway without even a backward glance.

'What's going on?' Arlo asked. 'Where's *she* going?'

'I'm not quite sure,' Jake responded. Had Isla said she was heading to the accident scene to assist the ambulance officers or was she going to the medical centre to help the GP?

'So what are we supposed to do?' Arlo shook his head. 'Nothing?'

The flashing beacon was a long way down the driveway now, about to turn onto the road.

But Arlo had a point. Jake wasn't about to sit here and do nothing when there were people out there who might need the kind of lifesaving medical skills he'd spent his life learning how to provide.

'We're going to help,' he said. *Whether Isla wants us to or not*, he added silently. 'Have you got your seat belt done up?'

'Yeah.'

'Good. Hang onto your hat.' The car took off with a slight skid as Jake put his foot on the accelerator.

* * *

Unbelievable!

Isla could see the headlights of Jake's vehicle behind her as she turned onto the main highway and increased her speed, heading north this time. He was keeping up with her but she knew these roads like the back of her hand and he was a stranger to the area. He shouldn't be driving this fast. He especially shouldn't be driving this fast with a child on board, but she had to concede that he was handling his SUV with the kind of skill she had come to expect from him in everything he did at work.

And…she couldn't deny that those skills might well be more than useful at an accident scene. A serious accident scene, she realised as she saw the flashing lights of both police cars and a fire engine blocking the road ahead. The firies had put a tarpaulin over the windows of a farm truck lying tilted into a stormwater ditch. Was that there to protect a trapped motorist from the weather? No…they wouldn't be left alone like that. It was far more likely to be screening someone who was beyond any medical assistance.

A mangled motorbike lay on its side, one bent wheel uppermost and the other jammed under the truck. Isla could see a crumpled body still wearing a helmet, also partly beneath the truck. A paramedic was crouched beside the patient and it looked as though he might be putting an IV line in. Or trying to. A hand came up as if the man was trying to escape the procedure, or was he simply pulling the oxygen mask off his face?

At least Jake thought to park his car on the gravel

shoulder of the road, far enough back to stop the boy being traumatised by seeing too much. He also left his hazard lights on to warn any traffic that might be approaching. Isla parked her vehicle side-on to add to the screening from any potential spectators that the ambulance was already providing. The fire engine was doing the same on the other side and a police car was blocking the road to the north, the blue and red flashes of its beacons reflecting on the canopies of nearby trees. They'd left enough of a space between them and the crash scene for the helicopter to land when it arrived.

It was still raining but not nearly as heavily as it had been. The last of any daylight was fading and the scene was noisy. Firies were shouting directions as they stabilised the wreckage, radios were being used and the man who'd come off his bike might be lying very still but he was screaming in pain. Isla opened the back of her vehicle and got a large backpack out that contained her airway kit, IV supplies and all the drugs she would need to provide adequate pain relief. A paramedic was crouched beside the man.

'Hey, Liam.'

'Isla. Good to see you. I've just lost the IV access, sorry.' Liam's gaze went over her shoulder as he stood up. Isla turned to see Jake right behind her and while she could have taken leadership of this assessment and treatment of a patient, she didn't want to. Jake was the person she'd want treating her in a situation like this and both she and this patient were lucky that he happened to be here. Liam was responding to the natural authority Jake always had and stepped back to let Jake crouch beside the patient.

'My name's Jake,' he said. 'I'm a doctor. What's hurting the most, mate?'

'My *legs*...' He rolled his head as another agonised groan escaped.

'We're going to do something about that pain in just a tick. Try not to move your head, okay?' He glanced up as he undid the strap of the helmet. 'Isla, can you help me get this off? I'll stabilise his neck. Liam, can you get a C collar?'

Isla carefully tilted the helmet back and forth, easing it off, while Jake kept the palms of his hands on the man's cheeks to keep his head as still as possible.

Liam handed a cervical collar to Isla to slip into place and then held his torch, shining it under the truck. Isla felt her heart sink as she caught sight of a lower leg that was so badly injured she couldn't tell if the foot was still attached. Jake had also followed the line of light. Then his gaze caught Isla's and the silent conversation was as fast as taking in a new breath. They needed to extricate him to see the extent of what they were dealing with and control any blood loss. Moving him was going to be complicated by the potential pelvic and spinal injuries he might have, but their first priority had to be dealing with the intolerable level of pain their patient was in as fast as humanly possible.

'What's your name, mate?' Jake asked.

'Dave.'

'Okay... I'm going to put a line in your arm so we can give you medication to take that pain away, okay?'

'*Please…*' he groaned. 'Just make it stop hurting…'

'We will, I promise.' Jake was leaning close to make sure Dave could hear him. 'We're going to take good care of you. I'll get Liam here to hold your arm still for me. And, Isla, can you draw up some ketamine and morphine for me, please?'

This might be a very different environment to work together in but Isla knew how fast Jake moved and she kept just ahead of him, able to hand him everything he needed to get the IV access inserted and secured and then double-checking the drugs she'd drawn up so they could be administered. Within only a few minutes, the cries of pain were muted and they were able to get an oxygen mask back on Dave's face and take a full set of vital signs.

'We need a back board,' Jake said. 'And have you got a pelvic binder available?'

'Yes,' Liam said.

'I want to see if the other leg is trapped.' Jake looked up to signal the fire officer in charge of his crew. 'How stable is the truck?'

'It's not going anywhere.'

Jake took Liam's torch and lay on his stomach to wriggle further under the wreckage.

'Who's inside the truck?' Isla asked.

'Pat Murphy,' Liam told her. 'Do you know him? Old guy who lives a bit north of here—must be in his eighties by now, with a beard like Santa Claus and eyebrows to match.'

Isla nodded, sad to hear that it was a local who would be missed in the community. Everyone always knew when Pat was in the supermarket because his retired farm dog, a lovely old border collie called Ben, would be standing sentry by the front doors.

'I went out to him when he had a heart attack last year,' Liam said. 'But there was no way he was going to give up his farm.' He shook his head. 'I suspect it was a medical event that caused the accident. He had his GTN spray in his hand. I'm thinking he might be the person they were waiting for in the medical centre.'

'Where's Ben?' Isla moved so that she could see the flat deck of the truck. There was a dog box on the back of the deck but the door had broken off and there was no sign of the dog and no time to go searching in the ditch.

Jake's voice was muffled but still clear. 'Left leg's not trapped but there's an open tibial fracture. Partial amputation of the right lower leg with ongoing blood loss.' There was an urgency in his tone now. They could lose this patient if they didn't work quickly enough. 'Slide the back board under him and I'll get his legs onto it.'

They could hear the helicopter approaching as they slid Dave out from under the truck. By the time it had landed between the police car and the fire engine and the crew were on their way to take over the care and transport of their patient, Jake had a tourniquet around the leg to control the bleeding and Isla had set up IV fluids and got them running into the wide-bore venous access.

The Auckland helicopter crew included another emergency department doctor who clearly knew Jake well.

'Might have guessed you'd find a way to get in on the action,' he said. 'What have we got?'

Jake filled them in succinctly as they made their own assessment of their patient. Within seconds, they were working together to apply a pelvic splint, top up pain relief and shift Dave carefully onto the helicopter's stretcher, packaged securely enough to ensure that no secondary injury to his spine or pelvis was going to make his condition any worse.

It was dark by the time the helicopter was ready to take off again.

'Take care, Jake,' the Auckland doctor said. 'Let's catch up properly soon.' Then he turned to Isla. 'You guys have made all the difference for us getting him back to definitive care fast. It's very unlikely that leg's going to be saved but you may well have made the difference in saving his life.'

Isla caught Jake's gaze. He was the one who'd really made the difference. Yes, she would have done everything she could with Liam's help but she could never have dealt with this scene so competently on her own. She wanted to thank him properly but he was turning away already. Looking towards his vehicle. Worried about his nephew?

Of course he was. The boy had been on his own for a good half an hour.

'Hope you're not going to try and head back to Thames tonight.' A police officer came up to them as the helicopter took off. 'There's been a big slip between Kopu and the Taparahi Bridge and the road's closed.

They've got a team there working on it but it'll be lucky if they've got it cleared by morning, I reckon.'

Isla turned back to Jake. She could help him find a motel or somewhere to stay overnight, perhaps? Maybe he hadn't heard the news. He was already striding back to his car.

The police would take care of Pat and his vehicle. Liam took the ambulance back to the station in Tairua. Traffic had been banking up in both directions and Isla needed to move her vehicle to let a single lane open to get cars moving again. She pulled off the road, however, when she got to the gravel area where Jake's car was parked, its hazard lights still blinking. She couldn't see him in the driver's seat. She couldn't see a child in the car either. With a chill running down her spine, she killed her engine and got out. It was only when she got away from the brilliance of her headlights that she could see the small beam of light from a phone torch.

She found Jake hunched beside a small boy who was sitting on the edge of the ditch, his arm around a medium-sized black and white dog.

'Oh…you've found Ben.' Isla held out her hand to the dog. 'Is he okay?'

'Ben?'

'Pat's dog. He would have been on the back of the truck. I imagine the dog box broke open and he got thrown out. Is he injured?'

'He's cold.' It was the child who spoke. 'He won't stop shivering.' Two dark eyes were looking up at Isla and it felt as if she was being blamed for the dog's misery.

'He's had a big fright,' she said. 'And he's lost somebody he loved very much so he'll be confused. And scared.'

She could see the way he tightened his arms around the dog.

'I'll look after him,' he said.

'There might be someone else who wants to do that, Arlo.' There was a wary note in Jake's voice. 'And I'm not allowed pets in my apartment in Thames. We might not even find a place we can stay tonight if we have a dog with us. We can't all sleep in the car.'

Arlo was still staring at Isla. 'You're my mum's sister, aren't you?'

'Yes. I'm… Isla…'

'That makes you my aunt, doesn't it?'

Isla didn't want to be an aunt. It was too close to being a mother and she could never be that again. She didn't want friends, let alone family members in her life. Because it wasn't safe.

She knew what it felt like to be staring into the abyss of losing the people you loved. And how terrifying it was to fall as the edge crumbled beneath your feet.

But that was where this little boy was right now, wasn't it?

He'd lost his people. And now he wanted to look after a frightened dog?

What would it have been like to find something solid and warm and…*alive*…when you'd hit the bottom of that abyss? Maybe it might make it feel as if life was worth living again?

Isla closed her eyes for what seemed like a long, long moment.

She opened them again to find three pairs of dark eyes fixed on her. Arlo's, Jake's and Ben's.

She let her breath out slowly.

'You'd better come back home with me,' she said. 'Just for tonight.'

Okay…

Jake had known that the woman he'd worked with for the last year or so was not exactly outgoing.

She was friendly enough. Great with patients and she got on well with other staff members but, while it was genuine, it was kind of a superficial friendliness. Isla Preston kept her distance—to the point where it felt as if she was firmly behind an invisible barrier. You could see an attractive woman in her mid-thirties or so, who was amazingly good at the job she did, but you'd never feel like you *knew* anything personal about her at all. Jake had no idea whether she had a partner or a pet or what she liked to do in her time off work or her favourite food or what kind of books or movies she liked. He'd never asked, mind you, but information like that was often dropped unintentionally into a conversation in a staffroom or with a patient.

Did Isla ever do or say anything unintentional?

Jake suspected that she didn't. There was a quietness about her. A sense of self-control. Isla was aware of everything that went on around her but she chose not to engage in things that were outside a professional realm. And now he'd discovered that she was living like a semi-hermit—in the most out-of-the-way place you could find and still be able to engage with civilisation.

No wonder she'd been so shocked when he'd turned up uninvited on her doorstep. He was quite sure she would have preferred to excuse herself after being involved in that accident scene and go back to her private refuge alone. He'd felt the internal battle going on behind her closed eyes. If she'd said anything that made it feel like she was still dodging any link to her sister's child he would have walked away from her right then and there and taken on the entire responsibility for Arlo himself.

But she hadn't.

Jake had no idea what the cause of the struggle was or whether she'd won or lost that battle but he did know that it hadn't been easy and he felt oddly proud of her decision. Or maybe it was the fact that she was including Ben the dog in the invitation that was giving him a glimpse of the real Isla Preston that had been so well hidden.

He wanted to see more. Because he had a feeling he might like the person she really was.

The rain had tapered off into a misty drizzle by the time they arrived back at the unpretentious house in the middle of nowhere. Jake looked at the row of outdoor footwear lined up between the front door and an old armchair on the veranda of Isla's home.

'Better take your shoes off, buddy,' he said to Arlo.

'It doesn't matter,' Isla said. 'There's no carpet inside.'

Arlo wasn't listening anyway. He was staring at the other side of the armchair where several surfboards were propped against the wall. Most of them were a lot taller than he was but there was a much smaller one at the far end.

It was another glimpse into the life of a very private person and Jake's curiosity went up several notches. Imagining Isla in a wetsuit, poised on top of a surf-board was…intriguing, to say the least. It would suit her, he thought. There was a gracefulness about the way she moved that would lend itself to the dance of balance that surfing a wave required.

'Do you surf?' he found himself asking as Isla opened the door.

She managed to dismiss a potentially interesting conversation in a single word. 'No.'

Jake took the hint. 'Come inside, Arlo.'

He didn't move. 'Is Ben allowed to come inside?'

'Sure.' Isla looked over her shoulder as she reached to turn on a light switch. 'But he might not want to. He's been a farm dog all his life.'

Arlo looked down at the dog. Ben looked back up at him with all the intensity he might have used watching a rebellious sheep that wanted to escape the mob. When Arlo moved, so did Ben. Jake stood back and watched them go into the house ahead of him and found he was having to swallow a bit of a lump in his throat. He could feel the bond of loss that was already there between a small boy and a dog who probably both felt completely lost.

The interior of Isla's house was a surprise. It was simple and rustic but it had a warmth that wasn't just due to the amount of exposed wood and the log fire that was still glowing behind the glass of its door. The big, well-worn table in the centre of the room might only currently have a laptop in the middle of scattered papers and notebooks with an abandoned coffee mug on one side but it looked as if it had hosted thousands of family dinners. Jake could almost hear the laughter and clink of cutlery on plates and smell something like a celebration dinner of roast beef with all the trimmings.

A wide window seat was piled with cushions and the windowsills covered with a collection of shells. There was a big couch that sagged in the middle, an old piano with photos on top of it and a whole wall of shelves that were so crammed with books some of them were lying sideways on top of others. The shelves were punctuated by three doors that led off this living, dining and kitchen area that spanned the whole front of the small house.

'Bathroom's the middle door,' Isla told them. She was scooping the papers and notebooks off the table. 'There are towels in the cupboard. Feel free to get cleaned up or change into dry clothes. I'll get the fire going properly again so we won't run out of hot water.'

Jake went back out to his car to get the bags that still had their airline luggage labels. When he came back inside Arlo was sitting on the floor in front of the log burner with Ben beside him. Isla was nowhere to be seen.

'She's gone in there.' Arlo pointed to one of the doors. 'That's her room. She said we can share the other room. It's got two beds.'

Jake went into that room to put on a dry pair of jeans and a tee shirt. He took his wet shoes to put beside the fire to dry and found Isla putting a cast-iron casserole dish on top of the log burner.

'It's some frozen stew,' she told him. 'We're lucky to still have our power on, but this is the best way to thaw and heat something like this.'

She'd changed her clothes too and was now wearing black leggings tucked into sheepskin boots and a soft-looking jumper that was also black. Her long dark hair, that Jake had only ever seen tightly braided, was loose and the damp spirals were a surprise. She had curly hair?

'Can I do something to help?' Jake offered.

Isla shook her head. 'I'm just going to peel some potatoes. It won't take long. I need to make some calls to our local GP and the police too and make sure everything's under control.'

'Okay.' He fished a tablet out of the side pocket of the small backpack he was holding. 'Have you got Wi-Fi?'

'Yes, of course.' A shake of her head made one of those long spirals of hair fall over Isla's shoulder. 'I know this looks like a holiday house.' She shrugged. 'Probably because that's what it's always *been*. Doesn't mean I'm embracing an alternative lifestyle.'

She kind of was, Jake thought. But he was distracted from setting up a connection for the device he'd bought Arlo in an airport shop. 'This is your holiday house?' he asked.

'My family's,' she corrected. 'But I've been living in it for a while. My grandparents built it. I had every school holiday here for my entire childhood.' She picked up a bag from the corner of the kitchen and started putting potatoes into the sink. 'It was a home when I needed one,' she added simply.

There was something in her tone that made Jake want to ask as many questions as it took to understand what that meant, but there was also something in her tone that warned him not to. He watched her open a drawer to find a peeler and then saw her throw a tentative glance towards Arlo.

'Your mum was a good surfer,' she told him. 'Much better than me. She could stand up on a board by the time she was three years old.'

'Yeah…' Arlo was staring at the flames of the log burner. 'She taught me when we moved to Cornwall.'

He was silent for a long moment but then turned to stare at Isla. His tone was accusatory. 'Why didn't you ever come and visit us?'

'I didn't know where you were,' Isla said. She put the peeler down and turned to give Arlo her full attention. 'I didn't even know that you existed. I lost touch with your mum more than ten years ago when she went travelling after *our* mum died. She stopped doing social media and I had no way of finding her. I sent letters to the last address I had but they got sent back.'

'That would have been about the time she met my brother, Troy,' Jake told her. 'On a kibbutz in Israel. I think they both gave up on technology at that point. I hadn't been in contact with Troy that much after I came to live in New Zealand, mind you. Or before that, really…but I went to visit when I was in the UK for a conference about five years ago.'

Isla turned her head sharply at the mention of the

same time period she'd been living in this house and Jake was startled by something in her eyes. Something dark, like fear. Or grief? It was a time stamp that was significant.

This house was significant. It was part of Arlo's family history and that gave it a place in Jake's life now as well. A couple of days ago, Jake hadn't felt any kind of personal connection to this woman who was no more than a colleague. Now, threads of connection were all around the three people in this house and he could feel them beginning to tangle.

He knew his world had changed forever the moment he'd made that vow to care for his orphaned nephew. Now another life was changing and Jake knew it wouldn't be happening if he hadn't gone searching with such determination. It made him feel that he had another duty of care, and he found himself making another silent vow.

Isla hadn't asked for any of this. She needed taking care of, too.

CHAPTER FOUR

ARLO WAS LOOKING a lot younger than his nine years.

He hadn't eaten much of the slow-cooked beef casserole and mashed potatoes Isla had served. His face was pale and a bit pinched.

'You don't have to eat that if you don't like it,' she told him. 'I've got some ice cream in the freezer if you feel like some dessert.'

But Arlo shook his head. He pointed to his plate. 'Can I give this to Ben?'

Isla nodded. 'I've got some raw meat thawing for him, too.'

'Might be time you got some sleep,' Jake said. 'It's been a pretty big day for someone who's travelled right across the world in the last couple of days—especially when they've been sick enough to be in hospital for weeks before that.' His brow was furrowed with concern. 'Are you feeling okay, Arlo? Not feeling too hot? Or like you're going to be sick?'

Jake reached out to feel Arlo's forehead with his hand and Isla felt the rejection herself when Arlo jerked his head out of reach. She was reminded that this was a new relationship for him with a traumatised child.

She also remembered that Arlo had needed dialysis in ICU and that he'd been born with only one kidney.

She waited until Arlo was tucked up in one of the single beds in the spare room, with Ben fed and on a blanket on the floor beside him, before she broached the subject with Jake.

'Is he still at risk of kidney failure?'

Jake made a noncommittal face. 'Most people can live a normal life with only one kidney, but Arlo needed some fairly major abdominal surgery to repair his liver and spleen and full recovery's going to take a while. He's also been dragged away from the only life he knows so that's enormously stressful too. He's going to need careful monitoring for any signs of failure, like swelling in his hands or feet, fatigue, fever, itchiness…' He shrugged. 'You know the list of symptoms as well as I do.'

'You got yourself tested, didn't you? As a potential donor?'

'Yeah.' Jake leaned back on the couch and closed his eyes. 'I failed the serum cross-match test so I'm not suitable. His body would totally reject my kidney.'

The tiny huff of sound made Isla think of the way Arlo had rejected his touch to see if he was running a temperature and she felt her heart squeeze in sympathy. She let her gaze rest on Jake's face a moment longer. He looked different away from work. Or maybe it just felt different being with him in a personal space. She was far more aware of him as a man rather than simply another doctor or colleague, that was for sure.

A very good-looking man, with his olive skin and dark hair and his facial hair that was somewhere between designer stubble and a full-on beard and moustache. He had crinkles around his eyes and mouth that suggested he liked being outdoors. Or smiling a lot? Yes… Isla had seen him smiling often enough when he was with patients, especially kids. She'd heard the compassion in his voice and had thought, just casually but more than once, that if she was sick or injured, Jake Hammond would be exactly the sort of doctor she'd like to have looking after her.

He wasn't smiling when his eyes opened and caught her looking at him though.

'That's the reason it was so important to try and find any other relatives that Arlo had,' he said. 'I found a detective who was able to search parts of the internet I'd never have been able to access. We found Sage's details and her medical history and the names of family members, including an Isla McGregor who was her older sister, and when we did a deep dive on that name we found that she'd married someone called Luke Preston.'

Isla could feel every muscle in her body tensing. What else had he found out?

'It seemed like far too much of a coincidence,' he said quietly. 'But there were a lot of articles in newspapers that came up with that name flagged.'

The silence was so deep it felt as if Isla was in danger of drowning.

Again.

She knew what he would have discovered. He might not have been sure it *was* her but the name Isla Preston would have revealed the newsworthy story of two young doctors from Auckland who loved the sea so much they had their own yacht. They'd gone sailing for a weekend with their three-year-old son, Max, and the family dog, an old golden labrador called Ollie, and the boat had struck some unknown object out at sea in the middle of the night. A partially submerged container that had fallen off a ship perhaps. Isla Preston had been the only survivor of the tragic incident, still clinging to some wreckage before finally being rescued more than twelve hours later.

He wouldn't have found what happened after that because she'd managed to keep her escape private, closing down her life in Auckland and fleeing to hunker down in the family's holiday home as she tried, desperately, to hold onto something worth living for. She'd discovered an even better escape eventually, losing herself in the pages of the stories she could create, but it didn't pay enough to cover all the bills so she'd finally taken on part-time work in the nearest hospital.

It was the empathy in Jake's face that almost undid her completely. At least he had the sensitivity to not say anything else that would be prodding not-so-old wounds. He didn't even need to tell her how sorry he was because she could *feel* that.

It almost felt like a physical hug.

Not that anyone had hugged Isla in the last five years. If anyone had tried to get that close, they would have found themselves being firmly pushed away.

But this felt different. As if Jake could understand that at the time she'd needed her sister the most, she hadn't had the strength or motivation to keep hunting for her because it was all she could do to survive herself.

'I was a lot older than my younger brother, too. Troy was six years younger than me.'

Jake's tone was almost casual—as if this might or might not be of any interest to Isla but it was worth offering as a safer topic of conversation.

'When our mother died, he was only eight. I was fourteen. They put us in different foster homes and there was nothing I could do about that. My home was okay. His wasn't, but we were in different cities so I didn't even know how bad it was until years later. When I left school I got a job and tracked him down and said he could come and live with me, but he was fifteen then and in with a bad crowd and already in trouble with the police. It didn't work out. It got worse.'

Isla was caught up in his story. She could only imagine how hard it had been, but she was impressed that he'd tried to take responsibility for his younger brother when he was still only a teenager himself.

'Troy got arrested for car theft and joy-riding and he got sent to a secure boarding school. He refused to see me when I tried to visit,' Jake continued. 'I put myself through medical school after that and then I lost touch with him completely after he was released.' He caught Isla's gaze. 'I thought he'd chosen not to include me in his life because I'd failed him when he was just a kid. I couldn't blame him for that so I didn't chase after him, but…it didn't mean I didn't care.'

She nodded. She knew how easy it was to end up losing touch with someone you cared about very much.

'My dad died while I was in my second year of medical school,' she told Jake. 'Sage was fifteen and Mum took her to live in Australia for a fresh start. We had sporadic contact and then it just stopped after Mum died.' Isla swallowed hard. 'I could have tried harder, I guess, but she could have found me if she'd wanted to and… I had a lot of stuff happening in my life.'

Like study and the stress of her first hospital jobs, then a husband and a baby and then her whole life being ripped away from her in one fell swoop…

Isla blew out a breath. She didn't want to talk about any of that. Neither did she want to open the can of worms that had been left hanging—that she could be a potential kidney donor for Arlo if he needed it in the future.

Arlo… Her sister's child.

Her nephew.

Family…

Part of her was so drawn to that it was terrifying. Because she knew how it could end.

How it *had* ended. Grief for her sister was trying to cut through the protection she'd painfully built, piece by piece, over the last five years, but it was still there. Just beneath the surface of the comfortingly numb layer that was thick enough to be able to cushion any unbearable emotion.

She'd lost her sister now. The last part of her family that she'd known and loved. That cushion of protection was helping her control how much this news was affecting her. She needed to control it enough to let it sift into her consciousness by degrees, if that was possible. She could cope with that. What she couldn't cope with was having another child steal her heart; it was as simple as that. She couldn't do it because she hadn't got past losing the last one.

It hadn't really sunk in that she'd lost her sister, had it? This was *all* too much…

Isla found herself getting to her feet. 'I'm pretty tired myself,' she said. 'It's not likely I'll get called out again tonight with the weather settling but I should get some sleep anyway.' Or at least shut herself away in her room, which might feel like an extra layer of protection. She waved an arm around the room. 'Just help yourself to anything you need.'

'Sleep well, Isla,' was all Jake said. 'See you in the morning. And…thanks for having us.'

Sleeping well hadn't been an option and Isla got up early to make herself a pot of tea. There was no point opening her laptop and trying to do some writing because she was too aware of not being alone in her house. Wrapping herself up in a coat, she took her mug of tea and her phone outside to check the weather forecast and reports on any road closures in place. It was still windy and cloudy but the worst of the rain seemed to have passed and she found that, while the trip would be slower than normal, the road was clear enough for her to be able to get to work.

Even better, Jake would be able to take Arlo and Ben back to his house and give her some time to work out how she was going to deal with this new complication in her life.

Or maybe not.

When she went back inside to put her mug in the

kitchen sink, she found Jake had made a coffee. He was standing in front of her bookshelves perusing the titles. The bathroom door was shut and Ben was lying outside it, so presumably Arlo was getting himself clean and dressed for the day.

Jake greeted Isla and then tilted his head towards the dog. 'What's going to happen to him?' he asked.

'When I spoke to our local cop last night, he said he was pretty sure that Pat doesn't have any family and that it might be hard to find a home for an older dog like Ben.' She raised her eyebrows. 'There are rescue organisations that can help, of course, but I got the impression that Arlo's kind of bonded with him. Would you want to adopt him if no one else comes forward?'

'I can't.' Jake shook his head. 'There's a strict "no pets" clause in my rental agreement. I don't even have room for Arlo, to be honest. He's going to have to sleep on the couch until I can make some changes in my living arrangements.' His look was very direct. 'Unless you could look after Ben while I look into finding another place for us to live?'

Isla shook her head. 'I can't look after a dog any more than I could look after a child. I'm either working or travelling back and forth.'

'You work part-time.' Jake sounded surprised. 'A lot less shifts than I do. You think it's going to be easy for *me* to take on the unexpected responsibility of raising a child? And maybe caring for a dog?'

Isla bristled at his tone. 'My hospital position is not the only work I do.'

'Really?' Jake sounded intrigued now. He was

watching her over the rim of his mug. 'What else do you do?'

Isla glared at him. 'That's none of your damned business.'

'Whoa!' Jake held up a hand in a gesture of surrender. 'Okay… I get the message.' He gave his head a small shake and put his mug down on the bench, turning to face Isla. 'So you're not prepared to help with Ben. Even a temporary shared care arrangement?'

'I can't.' Isla couldn't help her voice rising in self-defence. 'I'm not set up to keep a dog. Quite apart from the fact that I don't *want* a dog, there are no fences here. He might try and find his way home and get run over. That's not going to help anyone, is it?'

Jake folded his arms. 'And what about Arlo?'

'What about him?'

'Are you prepared to be involved in your nephew's life?'

'I…ah…' Oh, help…what could she say? Of course she was prepared to be involved. Part of her was aching to be involved but it was at war with a bigger part of her that was…terrified.

'He can't *live* here.' She knew she was sounding horrified but that was how she was feeling. 'Any more than Ben can. It's. Not. Possible.'

The sudden bark from Ben in the silence that followed her overly enunciated words was unexpected enough to make them both swing to face him. The bathroom door was slightly ajar.

'Oh, *no*…' Jake's words were almost a groan. 'Arlo didn't hear any of that, did he?' He strode towards the bathroom and pushed the door. Isla could see that the window in the small room was wide open, the metal arm that fastened it still swinging.

The look Jake gave Isla as he changed direction and headed for the front door was furious. Ben was at his heels and shot outside as soon as the door was opened. Jake ran after him and Isla followed, not even slowing down to close the door.

Ben was heading into the forest around her house.

'Where's he going?' Jake shouted.

'There's a track down to the beach.'

The thought that Arlo wasn't heading for the road was a relief. Or was it? After yesterday's horrible weather the surf would be huge and smashing over the rocks at each end of the bay. How dangerous would that be for a small boy who wasn't a hundred percent well and might only need to put a foot wrong to be in serious trouble?

What was even worse was that this was *her* fault. This poor kid had just lost both his parents and he'd been listening to one member of his only remaining family making it known that she didn't want him in her life—or that he wasn't welcome to live in her house, anyway. If she could have pulled those words back, she would do it in a heartbeat. Or at least explain why she had said them.

Isla looked sideways at the rough shelter that had racks holding the old kayaks that had always been a part of summer holiday fun when she was growing up. The closest they'd been to the beach for years was the windblown sand that made a carpet for dead leaves inside them.

Ben was a long way ahead now and barking loudly. Jake's voice was fainter.

'Arlo? *Arlo*…wait…'

Isla almost tripped over a tree root and the jolt was enough to make her change her mind about telling Arlo why she'd said what she had. She couldn't tell a nine-year-old boy that it was unbearable to be around him because he was almost the same age her precious son would be if he hadn't drowned and it would be like having a ghost in her house as well as her heart.

She couldn't even bear the idea of having a dog living with her because…because she'd watched Ollie drown…

How many times could a heart break and still keep beating? Isla had her hand pressed to the left side of her chest as she reached the sandy beach—as if she was trying to control the pain of the break. Jake was right in front of her and he'd stopped in his tracks, giving the impression he wasn't sure what to do next. Ben had carried on and he was now sitting, ramrod straight, beside the figure of the small boy who was looking out to sea, to the odd island that had a rocky base, tall steep sides and a bunch of trees growing on top like fluffy green hair. Arlo's fingers were resting on the sleek hair of Ben's head, between his ears, and Isla felt a kick in her chest at the level of her heart. Ben was exactly what Arlo needed in his life right now and there was only one right thing to do.

She walked past Jake and on to where Arlo was standing with the last foam of overexcited waves rolling over his bare feet.

'I'm sorry, Arlo,' she said to him. 'I didn't mean it. I *can* help look after Ben for you.'

He didn't look at her but she saw his fingers move, gently rubbing Ben's head.

'Can you get out there?' he asked a few seconds later. 'To that island?'

'Not in weather like this. And it's a bit steep to climb. It's more of a sea stack than an island. The swimming here can be good, though, and so's the surf—you just need to watch the tides and look out for the rocks. Sailors Grave doesn't have the rocks but the waves are wilder. This beach is the best to start with. Maybe you'll want to try out one of those boards one day.'

Arlo shrugged. 'Maybe…'

He turned back to where Jake was now within earshot. 'Can we go home?' he asked.

The relief on Jake's face was another thump in Isla's chest. He really, really cared about this boy, didn't he? His life was being turned upside down even more than hers right now. His relationship with his brother had been even more tested than hers had been with her sister but…he still *cared*.

Isla admired that.

Maybe she envied it, too. Because she'd lost the ability to feel that much?

'Let's have some breakfast first, mate,' Jake said to Arlo. 'Me and Isla have a few things to sort out—like how we're going to look after Ben until we can find a proper house for us.' He looked over the top of Arlo's head and his gaze was a challenge.

Isla managed to find a smile. 'Breakfast sounds like a plan. Do you guys like bacon and eggs?'

CHAPTER FIVE

'ALL GOOD?'

The glance into the rearview mirror was automatic. So was talking to the dog who was sitting in the back seat of Isla Preston's car, dammit.

Not that she was going to get attached to this animal. Even when she found the pair of dark eyes meeting hers in the mirror. Ben was in a harness with an attachment that clipped into the seat belt buckle. Isla was only too happy to comply with new legislation that made it illegal to have a dog loose in a vehicle because it meant that Ben couldn't sit with his head visible between the seats every time she looked down, like Ollie used to do, hoping to be noticed and patted.

'You can have the window down a crack, if you like.' Isla pressed the button on the armrest of her door and put the back window down a couple of inches. Another glance in the mirror showed Ben's chin tilted far enough for a black nose to be on the outside of the car, ready to catch any and all interesting smells.

He'd slept on the veranda last night on a perfectly comfortable blanket and Isla refused to feel guilty that she hadn't put that blanket in a corner of her bedroom. She wasn't the one wanting to adopt this dog who'd lost his person and the last thing she would want would be to wake up and find the dog on her bed. Being in the car with her was too close, in fact, but this was one of the arrangements she and Jake had agreed to yesterday morning over breakfast.

Ben would spend his nights at her place until they found a suitable property for what had just become a family unit for Jake Hammond, and a single-bedroom apartment was not remotely suitable. If he couldn't find a house to rent, he'd told both Isla and Arlo that he'd buy one. He'd been planning to do that as an investment, anyway.

Isla would take Ben to work with her and they would find a place to tie him up during the day. Jake would take him for a walk when he got a lunch break and Arlo would come and look after him after school. Because today was going to be his first day at his new school. Jake hadn't worked at the hospital yesterday—he'd been busy sorting school uniform, books and stationery, dog food and accessories like a harness and lead. He'd even introduced himself to local real estate agents. He'd looked beyond weary when he'd come to the hospital to drop Ben off to go home with Isla and told her that he'd be back on deck by eight-thirty a.m. tomorrow morning, as soon as he'd dropped Arlo off at school.

Isla was going in early this morning, having agreed to cover for Jake as much as she could for the next few days as he dealt with these first major changes in his life. They hadn't yet talked about what would happen on her days off or the coming weekend when Arlo wouldn't be at school, perhaps because there was so much happening, it was only possible to take one day at a time and deal with each issue as it appeared.

As she'd said to Jake yesterday, making sure they were out of Arlo's earshot this time, Isla was not going to dodge any responsibilities to her sister's child. They would work together and find solutions to any problems. Isla was relieved to find it was less difficult than anticipated to find a place to leave a dog while she was working. She spotted the enclosed pen as she walked past the back of the kitchens and spoke to someone who was only too happy, after hearing the story, to shift the recycling and rubbish bins to make room for a bereft dog, his blanket and a water bowl.

And then, finally, Isla could take a deep breath, walk through the doors of Coromandel Hospital's emergency department and step back, temporarily at least, into normality.

Sam looked up from the notes she was writing at the reception desk where one of the senior nurses, Laura, was on triage duty.

'Hi, Isla. How did you get on last night?'

Sam had been arriving to cover the night shift when Jake had turned up with Arlo yesterday to transfer Ben into her car and part of the handover of the day's patients who were still in the department had included a brief explanation that Arlo was Jake's nephew and now his responsibility and that she was helping out with the dog that had needed rescuing. She hadn't yet admitted her own connection to either of the developments that had turned Jake's life upside down and her response to Sam's query this morning was just as succinct.

'Fine, thanks. How 'bout you? Busy night?'

'Average. Back pain from a ruptured disc, non-cardiac chest pain, TIA who's been admitted for observation, elderly man with delirium due to a UTI and—' the list Sam was reading from the whiteboard was interrupted by a loud groan from one of the curtained cubicles '—and that's Tyrone. I strongly suspect man-flu but his chief complaint is chest pain so I thought I'd better put him on a monitor for a while and do an ECG and some bloods.'

Isla smiled. 'Give me two minutes to get my scrubs on and I'll take over. You should get home. You've done a long shift.'

Sam shrugged. 'We're all ready to help Jake. He's a bit of a hero, isn't he? Taking on his nephew *and* a rescue dog at the same time?' She exchanged a glance with Laura, who sighed.

'You'd think it would knock him off the top of Coromandel's most eligible bachelor list, wouldn't you? But I have a feeling it'll only make him more attractive. Just as well I'm happily married.'

'And I'm happily single,' Sam muttered. 'Husbands, kids and dogs do not feature in any of my life goals.'

Isla was already on her way to the changing rooms but she could feel her jaw muscles tightening. Forty-eight hours ago, like Sam, she would have been dismissing the possibility of including any of those things in her own life with just as much confidence. But she'd just spent a night with a dog and she had a horrible feeling she might be expected to spend her weekend with a kid. Maybe she should warn Sam about tempting fate.

* * *

By the time Jake came into work, Isla had taken Tyrone's history and examined him. She was wheeling the ECG machine into his cubicle when Jake came into the department. In his pale blue scrubs, his lanyard and stethoscope around his neck, he looked exactly as he always did at work.

So why did it *feel* so completely different?

Why on earth was Isla so aware of him? His bare arms. That tousled hair. Good grief, she could even catch a whiff of the soap or shampoo he must have used this morning. Something woodsy and masculine.

Or was that just Jake's skin?

He wasn't aware of the way her eyes widened in consternation because he was looking at the machine she was pushing as he walked towards her. She'd never really noticed how tall he was either, had she? Or that relaxed way he had of walking that suddenly made her think of cowboys in a movie, sauntering into a bar. Slightly desperately, Isla tried to make this proximity about nothing other than a professional interaction.

'I'm about to do an ECG and rule out an infarct and confirm a probable case of man-flu,' she told him.

Jake shook his head but he had a twitch of a smile. 'How did you get on with Ben last night?'

'Fine.'

'Where is he now?'

'Behind the kitchens. In the rubbish and recycling pen.'

'Right...' Jake blinked. 'I'll go and check that he's okay as soon as I get a break.'

It was Isla's turn to nod. She knew it was also her turn to show interest in his side of their new connection. 'How did Arlo feel about starting school?'

'Nervous as hell,' Jake said. 'But he was hiding it well. He's a brave kid.'

Jake was smiling as he peeled away to go and look at the whiteboard. He'd sounded proud of his nephew.

Their nephew.

Isla pushed the machine through the gap in the curtain around Tyrone's bed. 'I'm going to put some more sticky dots on your chest,' she told him. 'This takes a more comprehensive view of your heart than the one in the ambulance did.'

The curtain behind her rippled as someone went into the next cubicle and Isla had to refocus to find the correct position for the electrode in her hand as she heard the voice that confirmed it was Jake seeing the patient next to Tyrone.

What *was* it with this acute awareness of a man who'd only been a colleague until a matter of hours ago?

That was the problem, wasn't it?

He'd stepped out of his professional space and into her *personal* space. No wonder she was noticing such personal things as the smell of his shampoo and the rumble of his voice. It felt as if a locked door had been jimmied open and, as much as she wanted to, it was proving impossible to push it completely shut again.

Something was different.

Or maybe *everything* was different?

There was a connection now, between himself and

Isla, that had changed everything. No wonder she seemed wary of him today. Jake was feeling a bit wary of her, to be fair.

And that was making him so aware of her.

He kept catching sight of her, coming in or out of a curtained cubicle on the other side of the emergency department, that long braid of dark hair swinging as she turned her head. It made him remember the long spirals when it was damp and the glossy waves that flowed down her back when it got dry in front of the fire, later.

He heard the sound of her voice as she spoke to a paramedic who was transferring a patient to her care and snippets of what they'd shared about their dysfunctional relationships with their siblings came back to mind. Or, more pointedly, what they hadn't talked about which had been hidden in that casual line Isla had quietly uttered.

I had a lot of stuff happening in my life...

Jake was even more aware of that when a distressed parent ran through the doors of the department as they opened to let an ambulance crew out. She had a young child in her arms. Isla was beside the main desk, talking to Laura.

'*Help!*' the mother called. 'He *swallowed* it!'

Jake saw Isla's eyebrows rise sharply. 'What's he swallowed?'

'One of those button batteries. The ones that burn holes in their stomachs. Here...take him...*please...*'

She pushed the child towards Isla, who instinctively held out her arms to take the little boy, who looked about eighteen months old and was clearly aware of the stress his mother was radiating. He looked at Isla with wide, frightened eyes as if he knew he was in trouble and his bottom lip began wobbling. Jake walked swiftly to join them.

'Did you see him swallow it?' he asked.

'I saw him swallowing *something*. And he was using the remote control for the TV as a drumstick and he must have broken the battery case and…the battery was nowhere to be seen.' The mother had tears streaming down her cheeks and her voice was shaking. 'I looked *everywhere*. Is it true that it can kill a baby in less than two hours?'

Isla's tone was calm. She was heading towards the resus room. 'Don't panic,' she told the mother. 'We've got this.' She looked back at Laura. 'Can you get a radiographer on the way, stat, please? And we should have some honey in the staffroom. Could you bring that, please? And a teaspoon?'

'*Honey?*'

'It can slow down a chemical reaction,' Jake told her. 'And prevent injury.' He smiled at the woman. 'What's your little boy's name?'

'Leo…'

'And how old is he?'

'Sixteen months.'

'Come with us. Leo will be a lot happier if you can hold him while we check things out.'

Leo started crying as they all went into the resus room. Isla looked over her shoulder and caught Jake's gaze and he gave her a small smile, too. At least it was obvious that Leo wasn't showing any signs of airway obstruction from having a battery lodged in his oesophagus, which was the most dangerous place it could be. Saliva on the battery could trigger an electrical current and that could generate hydroxide, which caused alkaline burns. Leo's mother was right. The most serious complications, like bleeding out from a burn injury that was too close to a large blood vessel, *could* kill a child in a short amount of time.

Isla shifted her gaze to Leo's mother. 'Could you come and sit on the bed, please, and hold Leo? I want to listen to his breathing and check that he hasn't put the battery into his ear or up his nose. Has he been showing any symptoms? Like coughing or dribbling or vomiting?'

'No. But he was making faces as if he'd eaten something he didn't like and…and it can't have been the toast he was holding because he loves his toast.'

Laura appeared with the jar of honey and a spoon.

'Two teaspoons,' Isla instructed. 'We'll do that every ten minutes until we can rule out an oesophageal position by X-ray.'

'Monique's on her way,' Laura said.

'Can I look up your nose?' Isla asked Leo.

'*No.*' Leo shook his head firmly and buried his nose against his mother's arm.

'Would you like a spoonful of honey?'

He turned to look at the spoon.

'Yum, yum, yum,' Isla said, her smile enthusiastic. She held the spoon high enough that Leo tipped his head back to keep an eye on it. Jake quickly angled the overhead light enough to give them both a glance up his nostrils, where there was no flash of anything metallic.

Monique arrived to take a chest X-ray as Isla managed a quick look in both Leo's ears while he was licking his second spoonful of honey. Jake helped the mother put on a lead apron so she could hold Leo still and then he and Isla went to take more of the heavy aprons from the rack in the corner of the room. They stayed there to keep out of the radiographer's way as she got him into the best position to take the X-rays.

'We'll need to get him to a paediatric surgeon for endoscopic removal ASAP if it is in his oesophagus,' Isla said quietly. She hadn't bothered to tie the tapes on the side of her apron. 'That'll mean a helicopter ride to Hamilton or Auckland.'

'And if it's in his stomach?'

'He's asymptomatic. Could be a "wait and watch" situation but I'd like to be sure of the battery size first.' But Isla was frowning.

'What?' Jake asked.

'I'm not convinced he's swallowed it at all,' Isla said. 'If he was already eating his favourite thing, would he really want to put something else in his mouth?'

Leo started crying again as the last image was taken.

'He's sopping wet,' his mother said. 'I didn't think to bring any nappies with me. I just grabbed him and ran out of the house.'

'We've got nappies,' Isla told her. 'Laura, could you find one, please?'

Monique had the X-rays up on screen and both Jake and Isla went to look.

'No sign of the battery in the oesophagus,' Jake said. 'That's good.'

'Can you scroll down? Is it in the stomach?'

They were both watching the screen as they heard Leo's mother behind them.

'Oh… Oh, *no*…!'

They both swung round to see what disaster might be unfolding. Leo was lying flat on the bed, his nappy off, his mother holding it in her hands and staring into it.

Jake was there in a single stride. 'Oh…' he echoed. He was trying to hide a smile as he looked up at Isla. 'Guess what's in the nappy?'

'Why didn't I think of that? He used to hide things in his nappy all the time.' Leo's mother looked horribly embarrassed. 'I'm so sorry. I've wasted everybody's time, haven't I?'

'Don't be sorry,' Jake said. 'We'd much rather respond to a false alarm than not respond to something serious.'

Isla was nodding her agreement. And smiling. 'All's well that ends well,' she said. 'You did the right thing bringing him in.'

Jake saw how quickly her smile faded as she turned away, however, and it reminded him of how he'd always thought of her—as being distant. Unwilling to get involved with her patients, even.

Now he knew so much more about her, he was amazed that she was able to do this job at all, let alone do it as well as she did.

How old had *her* child been when he'd died?

How could she be so calm around other people's sick or injured children now?

Because she'd built walls that were a mile high around her personal life? Around her heart? Walls that he'd done his best to barge straight through by bringing Arlo into her life?

He needed to tread more gently, he decided when Arlo walked to the hospital after school finished, as they'd arranged this morning.

Jake was due for a break and took him out to play with Ben on the big grassy field where the helicopter landed if patients needed to be transferred to a bigger hospital—like they might have had to do for Leo earlier today if he'd needed specialist paediatric care.

'How was school?' Jake asked.

'Okay, I guess.' Arlo found a stick that he threw for Ben, who delightedly retrieved it to drop back at his feet.

'Not easy being a new kid, is it?'

Arlo threw the stick again.

'How are you feeling?' Jake asked. 'Not too tired? You can have a day at home if it's too much, too soon. I can always take a day off if I need to. Maybe I should get you checked out by the specialist in Auckland that I've lined up to keep an eye on your recovery.'

Ben dropped the stick again and was half-crouched, waiting for the instant the stick was airborne again.

'I need to go back inside again now,' Jake said, 'but you can play out here with Ben for a bit longer if you want to. When you've put him back in the pen, come through that door over there and ask the first nurse you

see to show you where the staffroom is. You'll need
to wait there until I've finished work for the day. We
need to find time to talk to Isla, too.'

'What about?'

'The weekend.'

Arlo threw the stick as hard as he could. Ben leapt
to catch it as it was spiralling through the air, which
made him grin. 'What about it?'

'Well… I've got to work on Saturday. I can't leave
you alone in the apartment when there's no school.
I can find someone to look after you, but maybe we
could ask Isla if it would be okay for you to be at the
beach with her for the day. Might be a lot more fun
than being stuck inside all day.'

'Would I have to stay the whole weekend?'

'Not necessarily.' That was something they needed
to talk about, wasn't it? Pushing Isla into more involvement than she could cope with might destroy any
chance of Arlo gaining a meaningful relationship with
his aunt in the future. 'I could drive you over and then
come and pick you up in the evening.'

'Where's Ben going to be?' Arlo asked.

'With Isla.'

Arlo nodded. 'Then that's where I want to be,' he
said.

CHAPTER SIX

ALEX WAS THE kind of person who got described as being complicated. Undeniably handsome with those sleek waves of dark hair and that neatly trimmed beard and moustache, he was highly intelligent, a dedicated professional when it came to his work, but he could also turn on the charm and bewitch anyone he chose to.

Riley never knew quite what to expect. She was in love with him, which coloured her judgement, of course, but there was every reason to admire him even if there were times when she had to confess she was more than a little afraid of him. He could make her forget any dark thoughts, however, the moment he touched her.

Oh, my goodness…

She had planned to talk to him as soon as they were alone tonight. What had gone wrong with that apparently healthy young man who'd come into the emergency department this afternoon with what looked like no more than a viral illness? Alex had taken bloods and put fluids up because he was dehydrated but he'd got worse so fast. Shaky, sweaty, confused and then… so aggressive. It was the closest Riley had been to a physical attack in a long time and it was Alex who'd pulled her out of harm's way. The bruise was already coming up on her arm, but knowing he cared that much about her safety more than made up for how rough he'd been. Didn't it?

'Get security!' he'd yelled. 'Stat!'

Only they hadn't got there in time and the patient had ripped out his IV line and vanished and the search had only ended when someone found him outside at the bottom of some concrete stairs, having a seizure that had resulted in the fatal head injury as his skull cracked repeatedly against the edge of the step.

But how could she start talking about work and these fatal cases that were increasingly bothering her when he was giving her 'the look'? When he did that thing where he put the pad of his finger on the middle of her forehead and then traced the outline of her face so gently that it tickled, as if he was holding a feather? She always closed her eyes, waiting for the moment his finger would touch her lips, because she knew what was coming next. His lips, on top of hers, his hands cradling her head now—kissing her so thoroughly her bones were melting and he would have to scoop her up into his arms and carry her to their bed and...

...and, dear Lord... Isla had to stop typing because she couldn't see what she was doing any longer. Because she was sitting here at her kitchen table with her head tipped back, her lips parted and her eyes closed. She could actually *feel* this sex scene she was about to write as if it was happening to *her*. Right this minute.

She could feel the spirals of desire wrapping themselves around parts of her body she hadn't bothered even thinking about for…years. She'd pretty much got to the point where she'd decided that she couldn't care less whether she ever had sex again in her life, but her body was telling her something very different right now. There was a void in her life that she was suddenly missing. Desperately. She wanted to be touched by another human. She wanted the world to stop turning for a little while as she was made love to. Slowly…passionately…

She was lonely. It was as simple as that.

She was lonely, but she was too scared not to be lonely because not being lonely meant that you had people in your life that you cared about and Isla knew exactly how dangerous *that* was. There was danger in her life now that she hadn't seen coming and she knew that protecting herself might be one of the biggest challenges she'd had to face yet in rebuilding her life.

Because, to her horror, she realised that it hadn't been the character Alex in her fictional story that she'd been thinking about as that scene was taking on a life of its own either. Good grief…when had she decided to give him some facial hair and brown eyes that crinkled at the corners when he smiled? Isla hastily deleted that new description that had slipped into her manuscript. Then she shut the lid of her laptop with more force than was necessary. She'd done enough for tonight, even though she'd been determined to make up for the time she wasn't going to get tomorrow, on her day off. Because Jake was bringing Arlo over for the day.

Isla gave her head a sharp shake. She did not want to think about Arlo. She especially didn't want to think about Jake. Or that weird awareness of him that had been growing ever since he'd turned up on her doorstep and upended life as she knew it. An awareness that had somehow snuck into her current book. What would her readers think if she wrote that entire scene that was still swirling in the back of her head? Or was it in her bones? They would be shocked, she was sure about that. Isla didn't shy away from having sex scenes in her story if there was a point to them but she didn't venture very far into the realm of what could be considered 'spicy'. Because hot sex was no longer a part of her own life, perhaps?

'Come on, Ben. It's bedtime.' Isla clicked her fingers and the dog was on his feet instantly. Why hadn't she put him out on the veranda hours ago? Had she been so lost in finally being able to get stuck into her writing or had it been kind of nice to have some company?

The sooner she was in her bed and sound asleep herself, the better. She just needed to make sure somehow that Jake Hammond wouldn't sneak into her dreams as well.

'So why's it called Sailors Grave Beach, then?'

'There's a grave. Do you want to see it?'

Arlo shrugged. 'Maybe.'

'We could take Ben for a walk. There's a track that leads from our bay back to Sailors Grave beach and it's not warm enough for many people to be around yet. A surfer or two, maybe.'

'Okay. This is kinda boring.' Arlo put his tablet down on the table. He eyed Isla's laptop. 'What've you been doing?'

'Oh…just a bit of editing on an article I'm writing. Nothing interesting.' Isla certainly hadn't gone back to that sex scene she'd started last night. When Jake had arrived with Arlo early this morning, she'd even glanced over her shoulder to make sure the laptop was closed. Or was it to check that there weren't wisps of steam escaping from the keyboard? It had been easy to avoid making direct eye contact with Jake, at least, because he was in a hurry to make the trip back over the hills and get to work. He'd lifted a hand to Arlo, thanked Isla for having him for the day, ruffled Ben's ears and then he was gone.

Isla had a kid and a dog in her space for the day and she was already feeling a tension that needed defusing. Getting outside for a while seemed like a very good idea. It was only about a thirty-minute walk to get from one bay to the next but it ended up taking so much longer. They picked their way in a companionable silence across rocks on the beach, with Arlo stopping to throw driftwood sticks for Ben or peer into the pools of water, touching anemones to make them close their frills or watching tiny fish dart beneath ledges to hide. Isla took her phone out to take a photo of the boy crouched beside one of the larger pools, Ben standing with his head level with Arlo's shoulder and both of them with their heads bent, staring intently into the water.

She sent it to Jake, having debated and then deciding against adding a text message. A response pinged back almost instantly. Two emojis. A 'thumbs-up' and then a smiley face. It almost felt as if Jake was on this walk with them and Isla found herself smiling as she slipped the phone back into her pocket.

The Sailors Grave memorial was inside a small, neat picket fence.

'So his name was William Simpson,' she told Arlo. 'He was a sailor on a British navy ship called the *HMS Tortoise* and he was twenty-two years old. He accidentally drowned in 1842 when the little boat they used to come to shore overturned in the surf. They buried him here and people have been looking after his grave ever since.'

Arlo looked fascinated. 'Why?'

'Do you know, I asked my dad the same thing, when he showed me the grave. He said it was more common for sailors to be buried at sea so it was a bit special to have an actual grave and his name and what had happened recorded. They must have really liked him, I think.'

'I read a pirate book where they buried someone at sea. They rolled him up in the hammock he slept in and sewed it up with rocks or something heavy at his feet so he sank fast when they tipped him off the plank.'

Isla blinked. This was the first time it felt as if Arlo was actually talking to her so what did it matter that the subject was gruesome?

So she nodded. 'You'd want them to sink fast. Otherwise, a shark might come and bite off something important. Like a foot.'

'Or his head.' Arlo's glance made it feel as if he was testing her.

Isla's lips twitched. 'That wouldn't be good.'

They turned away from the memorial but didn't turn back to go home. Instead, she followed Arlo and

Ben, who were heading towards the new beach of Te Karo Bay.

It was Arlo who broke the silence. 'Are there lots of sharks here?'

'I've never heard of one being seen. There's lots of fish, though. Nice ones, like snapper. And I've seen lots of little blue penguins.'

'No way.'

'Yes way,' Isla said firmly. 'I was swimming in the middle of summer once and a penguin swam right between my legs.' She couldn't resist stooping to pick up one end of a long, bleached driftwood branch. 'Your mum and I used to make teepees with sticks like this. We were allowed to just come and play on the beach all day by ourselves and we'd build a teepee and then sit inside it to have our picnic lunch.' She made a face. 'The sandwiches were always sandy but we were too hungry to care that much by then. Do you know, we both grew up thinking that was why sandwiches were called sandwiches? Because they had sand in them so often?'

That made Arlo roll his eyes but there was at least half a smile on his face. Something else had caught his interest, though. 'How do you build a teepee?' he asked.

'Well…you get long poles like this one and you stick the fat end in the sand as deep as you can and then put it at an angle, and when you get a few of them in place they start holding each other up.'

'Can we build one?'

Isla thought about the memories that would be stirred up by doing something she'd done with Sage so many years ago. She thought about all the work she needed to do on her book today. She thought about Jake, hard at work on the other side of the hills, doing the job that was still such an important part of her own life. And then, suddenly, the solution presented itself and she just stopped thinking about anything else to simply be in the moment and do something that required no more thought than what shape and sized driftwood poles she could find. For the next hour or more, she and Arlo searched for suitably straight branches and propped them up until they'd created a teepee with impressively solid walls. Arlo sat inside it when it was finished, with Ben beside him, looking out to sea. Isla took a photo of that too, but didn't send it to Jake.

Maybe she didn't want him to know that they'd been playing like a pair of kids on a beach. That she'd actually been enjoying herself.

He'd assume that she was bonding with her nephew, wouldn't he? He might expect more. He might have visions of them becoming so involved in each other's lives that they became some kind of family unit, even. If so, he was going to be disappointed. Isla didn't do bonding. The only way she could spend time like this with Arlo was to think about him as someone else's child. Her sister's. Jake's brother's. Jake's…

But maybe the answer to dealing with this was as simple as building the teepee had been. She could stop being afraid of the what the future might bring and not peer into the past too much and…just be in the present. To take each moment as it came, knowing that it would soon be a part of the past and there was no point in trying to predict what the future could be.

Okay, she shared a bit of DNA with this boy, but that didn't mean she had to try and be a substitute mother, did it? Or let him into her heart far enough to make it impossible to ignore the danger that he represented?

She glanced at the time on her phone. 'We'd better get back,' she said. 'You must be starving.'

'Yeah…' Arlo crawled out of the gap they'd left for the teepee door. 'Maybe we should bring sandwiches next time.'

Jake didn't get back to pick Arlo up until nearly six p.m.

'I stopped in Tairua,' he told Isla, 'and picked up some fish and chips because I thought I'd better feed Arlo before we drove home. There's plenty for you as well. They'll be getting a bit cold by now, though.'

'I can heat them up in the oven,' Isla offered. 'Sorry… I wasn't thinking. I could have met you at the Pauanui turnoff at Hikuai and saved you another hour's driving.'

'Hey, Uncle Jake…' Arlo raised his head from where he was sitting in front of the log burner, absorbed with whatever was on the screen of his tablet. 'We built a teepee on the beach.'

'Did you?' Jake handed the wrapped parcel of take-out food to Isla. 'That sounds cool.'

'It's what Isla and Mum used to do when they were kids. Isla took a photo. She sent it to me. Look—'

Jake hunkered down beside Arlo, scratched Ben's ears and looked at the photos of the teepee and the rock pools. He listened to Arlo telling him about the young sailor who'd drowned and realised that Arlo was talking

more and sounded happier than he had since…well…
Jake hadn't ever heard him sound quite this animated.

He stole a sideways glance at Isla, who was getting plates out of a cupboard to put on the table. Was it his imagination or did she seem slightly less uptight today? He wondered if it had been her suggestion for Arlo to call her 'Isla'. He could imagine that 'Auntie' might seem too familiar. Too close to having a child call her 'Mum'?

But how good was it that she'd spent time on the beach with Arlo? It gave him an odd catch in his throat and made him feel rather proud of her.

He cleared his throat as he straightened. 'Can I help? I didn't mean for you to be sorting dinner for us again.'

Isla handed him the plates. 'It's already sorted, thanks to you. You can put these on the table and there's cutlery in the drawer if you don't want to eat with your fingers. There's tomato sauce in the fridge and I've probably got some ghastly soft white bread in the freezer if you like chip butties.'

Jake could feel his grin spreading across his face. 'Chip butties are one of my favourite things,' he told her. 'You've made me a very happy man. Hey, Arlo— do you like chip butties?'

'Yeah…' Arlo was grinning too. 'As long as they don't have any sand in them.'

'Huh?' Jake threw a glance at Isla. He didn't get it.

'Inside joke,' she said, turning away and shaking her head.

The bookshelf on the other side of the long table caught Jake's eye as he set out the plates.

'Wow,' he said. 'You really like Tessa Townsend's books, don't you?'

Jake could sense the way Isla had frozen even from this far away. What on earth had he said wrong? 'I mean, I don't blame you,' he added. 'She writes brilliant medical thrillers. I've read more than a few myself.'

'Oh…?' The sound from Isla was vaguely strangled but she was focused on separating slices of frozen white bread to spread out on a plate to thaw. 'She's okay, I guess.'

Ah…so this was another 'no-go' area?

Fine. Jake stepped back from the brick wall he could feel between himself and Isla Preston. He headed for the fridge to find the tomato sauce and butter to put on the table. He didn't even try and make eye contact with Isla when he spoke.

'You don't happen to have some vinegar handy, do you? Or a bit of curry sauce?'

Isla gave a huff of what sounded like laughter. Or was it relief that the subject of a niche but popular author had been so decisively abandoned?

'I've probably got some gravy granules in the pantry. Would that do?'

Isla hadn't realised how hungry she was until they sat down to their meal. She'd given Arlo some baked beans on toast for his lunch when they'd got back from the beach but hadn't had more than a cup of coffee herself. The crispy batter around the soft snapper fillets was delicious. So were the thick-cut chips. She was a purist when it came to eating hot chips and only wanted a good sprinkle of sea salt on top of them, but she was watching in fascination as Jake gave Arlo a masterclass in making a chip butty.

'You need a good layer of butter on the bread.'

'Why?'

'Because that'll stop the bread going soggy when you throw on the vinegar and sauce. Or gravy. I'm going to put gravy on mine. Actually, I might put a bit of everything on mine.'

Arlo lined up a layer of chips with military precision on one slice of the buttered bread and reached for another one.

'Whoa…' Jake shook his head. 'You need a bigger chip to bread ratio there, mate.'

'What's a ratio?'

'How much of one thing you've got compared to another. The chips are the stars here, not the bread. Put as many as you can in and then squish the top piece of bread down to stick them together. The best butties are the ones that are almost too big to get into your mouth.'

It became a competition to see who could fit the most chips and condiments into the sandwich. And they were eyeing each other as they tried to hold their creations together while they took the biggest bite they could.

Isla could see the way they kept looking back at each other during the silence of dealing with overfull mouths. This was serious business and they were both entirely in the moment of butty appreciation, but she could see—and feel—what was going on that couldn't be seen. The bonding. The edging closer that was going to mean they would end up being the most important people in each other's lives.

For a heartbeat, it made her feel…left out.

Lonely?

No. This was actually good. Really good. Because it meant that Isla could stay right here, looking in from the outside.

Staying safe.

'I think,' Jake said finally, 'that this is *the* best chip butty I've ever had.'

He had a droplet of tomato sauce on the corner of his mouth and, for the life of her, Isla couldn't take her eyes off it. She wanted to lean over the table and remove it with her fingertip. What was worse, she could imagine herself licking it off her own finger.

'What?' Jake's eyes widened as he realised he was being stared at. 'Have I got sauce all over my face?' He rubbed his lips and the spot vanished.

Arlo hadn't noticed. He was trying to stop the contents of his butty falling out as he got ready to take another giant mouthful.

'It's pretty good,' was all he said.

'I might have to try one,' Isla said. 'Could you pass me a slice of bread, please?'

Arlo was yawning before he'd even finished his dinner and when Isla stole a glance at Jake she could see how tired he was looking as well.

'You don't need to drive back tonight,' she said. 'You're welcome to use the spare room again and go back in the morning.'

'Are you sure? That would be awesome, wouldn't it, Arlo?'

The warmth in Jake's eyes was nothing more than appreciation. So why was it that Isla could feel it seeping right into her bones? And why was she making a mental note to try and capture that feeling in her writing and give it to Riley to make sure that her heroine was going to remain under the spell of the man who was cleverly managing to kill off chosen patients that came under his care?

And why did it give her a strange feeling of pure pride that Jake Hammond had read her books? And liked them…

Arlo was sound asleep by the time Isla and Jake were washing and drying the dishes. Isla had turned a blind eye when she saw Arlo sneaking Ben's blanket into the spare room. The kind of palpable bond that was already there between the boy and dog might be the stuff of nightmares for Isla but she knew it was exactly what this lost child needed in his life right now and why would she want to interfere with that? As soon as Jake found a house for them to live in, close to the hospital and school in Thames, Ben would be living with them too and she knew he would probably end up sleeping on the end of Arlo's bed.

'Have you had a chance yet to look at what's available in the housing market?' she asked, putting the last plate onto the drying rack.

Jake picked the plate up to dry it. 'There are a couple of open houses tomorrow afternoon and I've got the day off. I thought it might be a good idea to take

Arlo with me and let him have some input into where he's going to live. One's an old villa with quite a big garden which might be good for Ben. If we get to keep him, that is.'

Isla had lived in an old villa once upon a time. With a lovely big garden for the dog. 'Sounds ideal,' she said. She focused on pulling the plug out of the kitchen sink. 'How was work today? Did you get the usual Saturday sports injuries in?'

'Sure did. Including the most dramatic one I've had so far.' Jake shook his head. 'I hope Arlo never wants to play rugby.'

'Head injury? C-spine?'

'Possibly both. Fifteen-year-old lad in by ambulance went into a scrum head first and was unconscious on the ground by the time they got the ball out and stepped back. Luckily, there was already an ambulance on the way for a badly sprained ankle. They did a great job of immobilising this kid but it looked like an obvious high cervical spine injury. Possibly complete at or above C5.'

'Was his breathing affected?'

'Not on the scene, but by the time they got to us he was clearly relying on intercostal muscles and his breathing was shallow. No diaphragmatic movement at all. He also had severe pain in his neck, headache and paraesthesia in both arms and hands.'

'Did you intubate?' Isla was wiping down the bench with a sponge.

'Yes. And we got onto organising a chopper at the same time to get him to the spinal unit in Auckland as fast as possible. He needed an ICU and Theatre available.'

'Must have been full-on,' Isla said. 'And then you've had hours of driving on top of that.' She turned to dry her hands but found that Jake was still holding the tea towel.

'It was worth it,' Jake said. 'To see how happy Arlo was looking. And maybe I'll get to go and see this teepee before we head back to town in the morning.' He was holding her gaze but he must have noticed her dripping hands because he offered her the tea towel.

Isla didn't respond. She took hold of the tea towel to dry her hands, only to find that Jake wasn't letting it go.

'Thanks for that,' he added softly. 'And for that photo you sent me of him and Ben looking into the rock pool. I got it just after the chopper took off with that lad and his father who was so desperately worried and… it felt like a little bit of balance had been restored in the world. That there were still good things out there.'

His quiet voice was a rumble of sound that flowed over Isla and made her look up to watch his lips moving. She could feel the warmth and shape of his fingers through the thin fabric of the tea towel and when she lifted her gaze to his eyes she found she was completely caught.

She could not look away. She could still see his lips in her peripheral vision and, oh, help…she suddenly remembered that drop of tomato sauce on his face and that shocking urge to remove it with her finger and taste it herself. She felt the tip of her tongue go to the corner of her own mouth, as if she needed to make sure she didn't have any visible sauce on her skin.

She saw Jake's gaze flick down and knew he'd seen what she was doing and then it felt as if she'd stepped into the pages of her manuscript that she'd abandoned last night because her physical response to what was happening in her imagination had become so over-whelming. She wasn't the only one who'd somehow stepped into that fantasy though. She could feel that Jake was right there with her.

Isla still couldn't look away.

Neither could Jake.

It was inevitable, wasn't it? That one of them—probably both of them—moved. In slow motion. Easily slow enough for either of them to duck away and stop it happening, but it was utterly obvious that they both wanted it.

They wanted their lips to touch.

They needed to know what it would be like to kiss each other.

It was just a kiss. Soft. Slow. Wordless, both before and afterwards.

It simply happened. A kiss like no other she had ever felt—or had she just forgotten because it had been too long? No…this was definitely something unique. So tender, so heartfelt and so beautiful it almost brought tears to Isla's eyes.

And then it was over.

It only took a matter of seconds, but apparently that was long enough to change everything.

CHAPTER SEVEN

OF COURSE THAT kiss shouldn't have happened.

The very last thing either Isla or Jake needed was another complication in their lives.

So, by tacit agreement, it seemed they were both going to choose to ignore it. They'd both been a bit stunned in its wake so it was no surprise that they'd just left it hanging a little awkwardly in the air and had gone into their separate bedrooms and shut the doors. Arlo was awake early the next morning so they weren't going to say anything that he might overhear and Jake got his wish to go and see the driftwood tee-pee before they drove back to town in time to go and look at houses for sale.

But now it was several days later and still nothing had been said. If Jake was still thinking about that kiss as much as Isla was, he was managing to hide it very well. Their interactions at work since then had been completely professional, but now they were heading towards another weekend where Arlo wouldn't be at school and he apparently wanted to stay with Isla and play on the beach with Ben, and that would mean Jake would be there at least some of the time and…

…and maybe that was why Isla was becoming even

more obsessed with that damn kiss. She had also given Alex and Riley what she suspected was the greatest sex scene she'd ever written but wonder whether she was going to let her editor, let alone anyone else, read it was enough to bring a flush of colour to her cheeks and a warmth to other parts of her body that were—rather disconcertingly—coming increasingly back to life.

They were both on duty in the emergency department of Coromandel Hospital this morning and they were both required in the resuscitation area when an ambulance crew came in with a seriously unwell man in his late forties.

'This is Steve. He's been short of breath on exertion since yesterday but deteriorated over a short period of time this morning. Respiration rate of forty on arrival, heart rate one twenty and an oxygen saturation of ninety-two percent on room air. No cardiac history.'

Isla could hear the high-pitched whistle of obstructed airways without any need for a stethoscope and found she had to deliberately close off the part of her brain that she used for her writing, along with any reminders of her invented scene of a fatal asthma attack. To her horror, with Jake close enough for their arms to brush as they transferred this patient to the bed in the resus room—'On my count. One, two, *three*…'—she also had to shut down the blurred boundaries between Jake and her fictional character Alex in terms of sexual attraction.

And…that *sex* scene.

Okay, that made it easy. Isla slammed the mental lid back on that can of worms. She put the back of the bed up to help their patient breathe more effectively and switched the tube connection to the oxygen mask from the portable cylinder from the ambulance to their piped overhead supply. Laura was clipping an oxygen saturation monitor onto a finger and then swiftly wrapped a blood pressure cuff around Steve's upper arm. Jake was quizzing both the ambulance crew and their patient, who was shaking his head to every question so far.

'Any chest pain?'

'Any fever or chills?'

'Do you have a history of asthma?'

'Any recent trauma to your chest?'

'Have you lost any weight recently?'

'We've got bilateral JVD,' Isla told Jake as she turned up the flow of oxygen. She was waiting a moment for Laura to attach ECG electrodes before using her stethoscope to listen to both lung and heart sounds. Distension of the jugular veins on both sides of the neck was a sign that something could be very wrong with the ability of Steve's heart to pump blood normally. 'Heart rate one twenty-four, respiration rate thirty-six, BP one ten on seventy and saturation is ninety-four percent on high flow oxygen.'

Jake gave a quick nod to acknowledge the information of less-than-optimal vital signs. He was also watching the ECG trace settle on the screen.

'Low voltage QRS complexes,' he commented. 'Laura, could you grab the bedside ultrasound, please? I'd like to do a TTE.'

This time, Jake caught Isla's gaze and she could feel the laser-sharp focus he had on their patient. He wanted to do a transthoracic echocardiogram, which was an ultrasound test for cardiac function, and she could almost see the list of potential diagnoses floating over his head. Cardiac tamponade was high on the list at the moment and a collection of fluid around the heart that could be causing these signs and symptoms and be enough to stop effective cardiac and respiratory function could be due to a variety of causes, like a lung malignancy, an acute infection or something even more serious, like a cardiac rupture after a 'silent' heart attack that had gone undiagnosed in the last week or two.

Minutes later, when she glanced up, having taken the first blood samples to go to the lab urgently, she caught the profile of Jake's face as he watched the screen intently, one hand guiding the cardiac wand on the chest wall to get the images of Steve's heart and its movement.

'There's a large effusion,' he said. 'Along with the right ventricular collapse during diastole, it's strongly suggestive of a tamponade.'

'What's that?' Steve's voice was muffled beneath the oxygen mask. 'Doesn't sound good.'

'It's a build-up of fluid around your heart. It creates pressure and makes it difficult to do what it's supposed to do and pump blood around your body. That means less oxygen getting where it needs to, so it affects your breathing as well.'

'I don't feel so good,' Steve said, only seconds later.

He wasn't looking good either. Isla noted the beads of sweat on his forehead, deathly pale skin and the way his eyelids were fluttering shut. An alarm sounded on the monitor as his heart rate increased and his blood pressure fell.

'He's crashing.' Her voice might be calm but she could feel the claws of panic digging into her chest as she reached to feel for a radial pulse.

Something made her look up as she did so, however, and she found Jake's steady gaze on her.

He didn't have to say anything out loud. The reassurance was there.

You know what to do, Isla. You've got this... We've got this...

Several things needed to happen very fast if they were going to save this patient, but if Isla had had any doubts about whether she was confident to cope with such a tense situation she was very wrong.

Perhaps wanting her to know how true that was made Jake decide to step back and watch her swing into action as she silently accepted the lead role in this life-or-death drama. There was no time for other investigations or a consultation with an interventional cardiologist from a bigger hospital. If the fluid wasn't removed from the chest, Steve was going to go into irreversible shock and die. Moving him to Theatre wasn't an option either, but resuscitation areas were well set up to become impromptu operating theatres. A sterile tray was set up and Isla scrubbed her hands at the sink before getting gowned, gloved and masked. Jake helped Laura prep the skin and drape Steve's chest, keeping a close eye on all the vital signs being monitored.

Isla held the plastic-wrapped ultrasound probe in one hand and a syringe full of local anaesthetic in the other. Jake could see that she was putting some local into the space around the heart as well, to ensure that the final part of this procedure where the fluid was sucked out and a drain left in situ was as painless as possible. Her hand was steady as she inserted the cannula, her gaze fixed on the monitor to navigate past an artery that was a pulsing red blotch on the screen very close to the moving shape of the beating heart. He could see the tip of the needle clearly as it entered the narrow fluid-filled space surrounding the wall of the heart.

He saw the way her eyes narrowed as she adjusted the lens of her focus to no more than the task she had in front of her and, just for a split second, Jake was captured by the way she was radiating her determination to succeed with her entire body.

The intensity of that focus and skill, along with such an obvious determination to succeed was…

…well, it was bone-meltingly sexy as far as he was concerned, that was what it was.

It was also a very unprofessional thought to enter his head, but it was becoming disturbingly familiar when the aftermath of that ill-advised kiss should have worn off by now. Yes, it had happened, but Isla had seemed just as happy as he'd been to pretend it *hadn't* happened. Possibly even happier. He'd done his best to put it out of sight and out of mind. But it simply wasn't working, dammit.

It was only for the tiniest blink in time but Jake knew he was nowhere near forgetting about it. Thanks to its frequent appearance, he could also be sure that he would be spending more time thinking about it in the very near future. Wondering who had actually initiated the kiss.

And whether it was going to happen again…

But not now, even if his supporting role allowed him to appreciate everything he was seeing. Like the precision with which Isla was inserting a guidewire into the cannula and then a catheter over the guidewire, frequently shifting the ultrasound wand to check the position of the tip. She attached a three-way plug to the end of the catheter and used a large fifty mil syringe to suck out as much of the effusion as she could.

'Blood pressure's coming up,' he reported. 'Heart rate's dropping.'

'I'm feeling a bit better,' Steve said. 'Like I can breathe again.'

'Good.' Isla closed off the valves and secured the line with tape and a clear sterile dressing, leaving the pigtail catheter in place to allow for continuing drainage. 'You just rest for a bit, Steve. We're going to arrange transfer so that we can get you in front of a specialist. When we find out what's causing this, we can try and make sure it doesn't happen again.'

Isla was only working a half shift today and Sam came in to take over at lunchtime.

'I saw the helicopter coming in to land,' she said. Her sigh was one of disappointment. 'I've missed a bit of excitement, haven't I?'

'You did,' Jake told her, looking up from the notes he was writing at the triage desk. 'Including a masterclass in managing cardiogenic shock by dealing with a tamponade.'

'Ooh… I've only done that on manikins on training

courses. Was it as dramatic an improvement as I've heard it can be?'

'She saved his life,' Jake said simply.

'It was a team effort,' Isla said. 'It was Jake who did the echo. He could have done the pericardiocentesis just as easily as I did. Anyway…' she adjusted the strap of her shoulder bag '…I'm going to head off. I've got a dog who needs to stretch his legs before I drive back over the hill.'

'Mind if I come with you?' Jake glanced at his watch. 'I'm due for a break and I could do with some fresh air.' He raised an eyebrow at Sam. 'You happy to hold the fort for twenty minutes? Laura will fill you in on our patients, but there's nothing of any great concern currently.'

'Of course there isn't,' Sam muttered. 'Yeah…get out of here and get your fresh air.'

Ben was delighted to be let out of the recycling bin pen. Isla didn't bother clipping a lead to his harness. She knew by now that this dog was not going to leave her side unless it was with an invitation to chase a stick or a ball. She wasn't quite as delighted as Ben, however, as they set off to cross the field where the helicopter had touched down briefly to whisk Steve off to the nearest cardiology department. She had the feeling that fresh air wasn't the real reason Jake had wanted to share this walk.

She was proved right almost immediately.

'I've got something I want to show you,' Jake said when they were halfway across the grassy patch. 'One of the houses that Arlo and I went to see last Sunday.

We had another look last night and I'm thinking of putting an offer in. It's only five minutes' walk across the road from here.'

'Oh…that's great.' Perhaps the end of her being a reluctant dog-sitter was closer than she had expected. Isla looked down to find herself catching Ben's gaze and it felt as if she could almost read the dog's thoughts.

Don't pretend you don't like having me around. You just don't want to admit it and that's okay. I still love you…

'Even better, it's empty at the moment,' Jake continued. 'I could probably get a really short settlement date and be in within a couple of weeks.'

They crossed the road on the far side of the paddock and then headed for a tree-lined avenue with old houses and big gardens on either side. Lovely villas that were over a hundred years old, with bay windows and stained-glass fanlights and verandas with wicker chairs that overlooked the mature trees and well-kept lawns bordered by gardens full of rose bushes and flowers. The one Jake stopped in front of even had a white picket fence with wrought-iron gates.

He couldn't have known how similar it was to the gorgeous old house that had been the family home she had left behind in Auckland five years ago. He clearly sensed that Isla was struggling, however.

'Are you okay?' he asked quietly.

Isla blinked fast. She wasn't going to cry. Why would she when she'd run out of her lifetime supply of tears years ago? She managed to nod in an attempt to convince both Jake and herself that she was fine.

'I love villas,' she said, but then she had to clear the catch in her voice by clearing her throat. 'This is… very like the house that Luke and I bought in Auckland, that's all. We even had an oak tree in our garden with a…a baby swing just like that one…'

There was a moment's shocked silence and then Jake swore under his breath. 'I'm *so* sorry, Isla. I wasn't thinking…'

'You're thinking about exactly what you need to be thinking about,' Isla said. 'And that's Arlo. Thank goodness he's got you to do that,' she added. 'Because I'm not doing a great job of it, am I?'

She had to blink hard again. How weird was that? When she'd hit rock-bottom in her grief all those years ago she'd been so sure that the door was closed on the part of her life where her heart was capable of feeling the kind of love—and pain—that could create tears.

Mind you, she'd been just as sure she'd never be interested in sex again either and the way Jake was looking at her right now, with that softness that suggested empathy rather than pity and a gleam that was contradicting her admission that she wasn't being the person Arlo needed her to be was, oh, dammit…it was taking her straight back to the feeling that kiss had given her.

An affirmation of a part of her that was almost forgotten. Of being a woman. Of being desirable…

She wanted him to kiss her again. Right now.

'Hey…' She tried to make her tone light. 'It's a gorgeous house and it's not as if I have to live in it. It's perfect for you and Arlo. And Ben will absolutely love this garden.'

'Ben absolutely loves your beach,' Jake countered. 'And so does Arlo. I'm sure we're going to find a way to make this work—for both of us.' His face scrunched into something close to a grimace. 'And this might be a good time to apologise for…you know…what happened the other night. I hope you don't think I was hitting on you.'

The disappointment that a kiss wasn't in her immediate future was balanced by the way Jake was taking responsibility for initiating that kiss. It felt as if he might be trying to absolve her of any guilt she might be entertaining in betraying a memory, perhaps? She liked that.

'I was hoping the same thing,' she said. 'That you didn't think I was hitting on *you.*'

The corner of his mouth lifted. 'I'm almost always the one who does the hitting,' he said. 'And then I back out before anything gets remotely serious because I'm phobic about relationships. I turned over a new leaf when I moved here, though.' That one side of his mouth curled wryly. 'Thought I'd better not undermine my reputation in a small town. You never know who you're going to meet in the local supermarket, do you?'

Isla wanted to ask why he had a phobia about relationships. Had he had a marriage end badly or had someone broken his heart into too many pieces in the past?

Not that it was any of her business. It was enough to know that there had been nothing significant in that brief kiss they'd shared. That it had simply been an intimate touch between two people who had no one else in their lives to provide it. That it had probably been such an insignificant occurrence in Jake's life he hadn't given it another thought. Until now.

She should be relieved. She *was* relieved. That pang of something beyond mere disappointment—feeling hurt, even?—was fleeting enough to be easily dismissed. This was like that blip of feeling left out when Jake and Arlo had been bonding over chip butties. When she gave it a little more thought, she could see it from an entirely different perspective. She didn't want significant.

She wanted *safe*.

'I have a reputation to uphold, too,' she told him. 'People think I'm a bit weird. A loner. A bit of a recluse, in fact. I don't think anyone other than you knows the reason I went to live alone at the beach. It's history now.' She bit her lip. 'I'd rather it stayed that way. It's not going to change—I'm never going to even want to try and replace what I lost because I know it's totally impossible but...' she pulled in a quick breath '...I'm not going to walk away from Arlo either. He's the only family I'm ever going to have now.'

Jake's smile was as soft as his glance this time. Had he noticed that Ben had nudged her hand with his damp nose as if he wanted her to remember that a dog could be part of a family, too?

'You won't have to even come into this house if you don't want to,' he said. 'And I'll never breathe a word of anything you'd rather people didn't know. But...'

Isla's felt a prickle of something run down her spine. Fear?

Hope?

'But…?' The single word was no more than a whisper but Jake heard it.

He glanced over his shoulder in the direction they'd come from, as if his thoughts were already turning back to work because his break was over. Then he shrugged and caught Isla's gaze again. 'I guess I just wanted to say that I think, given what you've been through, you're doing a great job as a brand-new auntie. And…'

His eyebrows lifted slightly, creating a crease on his forehead. Was he second-guessing whether to say what he was really thinking?

'And…?' she prompted.

'You don't need to worry about me kissing you again,' he said. 'I don't know why it happened and I'm sure Arlo would think it was completely gross that his auntie and uncle would even think of doing something like that, but… I guess… I like you, Isla Preston. I've never had the chance to get to know you, but I'm starting to like you a lot.'

'Oh…' Isla hadn't expected that and it gave her a lovely fuzzy sort of warm feeling inside. It also made her start walking back to the landing field and the hospital and the car that would take her to safety many miles away from Jake, but she couldn't resist a peep over her shoulder. 'I like you too,' she admitted.

She walked faster. Maybe she imagined the words she thought she heard Jake mutter behind her.

'I liked that kiss, too…'

CHAPTER EIGHT

JAKE'S PURCHASE OF the old villa close to the hospital became unconditional as soon as building reports and a valuation were completed, and suddenly he found himself having to furnish what was going to be a family home—something he'd never even contemplated doing.

'Where do I start?' he asked in the staffroom, looking up from the message he'd just received on his phone. 'I can go and collect the keys from the estate agent when I leave work but…it's an empty house. I don't own a single piece of furniture!'

'Go online,' Isla advised. 'If you buy a heap of stuff from one of the big home stores in Auckland, I'm sure they'd be more than happy to deliver it all within the next day or two. Just start with the essentials like beds and linen and a couch and table and kitchen utensils and crockery.' She scrunched up her nose. 'You're right, it is a lot.'

'It's not just about *things*,' Jake said quietly. 'I want it to feel like a home. Like your place does, Isla. It's so full of… I don't know… Maybe it's got something to do with the fireplace or all those books, but the feeling you get every time you walk in is like someone giving you a hug. And saying that you're welcome. I want Arlo to feel like that when he walks through the door into our house.'

'Aww…' Laura was making a toasted sandwich at the bench. 'That's such a beautiful thing to say.' But she gave Jake a curious glance. '*Every* time? Is there something we've been missing?' She was trying not to smile. 'And there I was thinking you two were happily single.'

Jake gave Isla an apologetic look. 'Sorry,' he mouthed silently.

She gave her head a tiny shake in response, telling him it wasn't his fault. 'There is something you don't know,' she told Laura. 'But it's not what you think. The connection is Arlo.'

'Jake's nephew?'

'Yeah…he's actually my nephew as well.'

Laura's jaw dropped. 'What the heck…?'

'Long story,' Jake said. He wanted to take the spotlight off Isla somehow. He knew how fiercely she guarded her privacy. He knew why she needed that protection from the pain that someone poking around in her past could cause.

'My brother ended up as Isla's sister's partner, but neither of us had the slightest idea until I had to go back to the UK after that accident.'

But Laura didn't seem to be listening. She was staring at Isla. 'I didn't even know you had a sister.'

'No…' Isla seemed to be fascinated by how much coffee was left in her mug. 'Unfortunately, I lost touch with her a long time ago. I wasn't really trying to hide the fact that Arlo and I are related. I've just been…'

Jake saw the way she swallowed hard. 'Trying to get used to it,' he put in. 'Like I am. And Arlo. We've all had our lives tipped upside down but the focus has been to try and give Arlo a place to call home again. So now I have a house. And I have to buy a lot of furniture.' Maybe changing the subject was the best way to handle this for the moment for everybody. Especially Isla. He swiped the screen of his phone to open a browser. 'What's the biggest and best home store in Auckland?'

Jake made the most of snatches of time between the flow of patients that came into the emergency department that day to show Isla the items he was considering and to ask for her advice.

'What size bed should I get for Arlo? A single? A king single?'

'He's going to grow fast and he might turn out to be as tall as you are. He'll probably end up having Ben sleeping on the end of his bed, too. I wouldn't go any smaller than a double.'

'Okay. And I might get a bigger one for myself. A queen or a king.'

'Oh?' Isla's voice sounded a little strained.

Oh, help...did she think he was revealing something about his intended love life? That he might want to go back to the 'love 'em and leave 'em' trail of female companions that he'd hit on in his past?

She couldn't be more wrong.

He'd been serious when he'd said he wanted to create a home for Arlo. A family space.

'Just in case they both decide to come and bounce on

me,' he added hurriedly. 'Like I've seen kids and dogs do in those family type movies.' He scrolled down the page on his screen. 'What about duvets and pillows?'

'You'll need them,' Isla agreed. 'Go for a size bigger than the bed. That way, there's enough to hang over the edges. Have you chosen a washing machine yet?'

'No...' He wasn't going to get the chance to add one to his cart right now either. Sam was poking her head through the staffroom door.

'I could do with a hand. We've got an eighty-year-old on the way in by ambulance with a fractured neck of femur, a guy in his fifties with central chest pain in the waiting room and one of the local tradies is apparently coming in by car with a tea towel wound round where he's had a go cutting off his arm with a bandsaw.' Sam looked more than happy with the influx of patients about to hit the department. 'I'll take the lacerated arm unless one of you guys wants to fight me for it?'

'It's all yours,' Jake told her. 'Isla, shall we assess the chest pain together until the NOF arrives?'

'Sure.'

It looked as if Isla was also more than happy to step back into an entirely professional arena and Jake was reminded that it wasn't simply her personal life being massively disrupted by recent events. Now that the cat was out of the bag about her connection to Arlo and—by default—himself, her professional life was going to change as well. People would know more about her. They might be curious enough to uncover things about her life prior to her starting to work in a smaller regional hospital. The refuge of her privacy was being breached. Had she healed enough in the years since the tragedy to be able to cope with it?

He hoped so.

But what was *he* thinking, trying to get her advice on how to furnish an old house that was a tangible reminder of a life she had lost—one that had been so important she never wanted to even try replacing it?

He ordered a washing machine and a dryer after he'd left Isla starting thrombolysis on the man whose blood tests and twelve-lead ECG confirmed that he was having a heart attack and helicopter transfer to a catheter laboratory was going to be delayed due to the major response needed for a three-car pile-up on the main state highway near Hamilton.

When X-rays had demonstrated that tripping over her cat had resulted in a fracture for eighty-year-old Norma, who was going to need hip replacement surgery, he made her comfortable with an effective dose of morphine and left her in the care of the nurses until transport by road could be arranged. Sam had gone into Theatre with the hospital's general surgeon to repair a gash from a circular saw that had reached the bone of the young builder's forearm, but Jake had enough time to add pillows, duvets, sheets and towels to an order that was already past the level where free and fast delivery was promised.

What else did he need? A kennel to go on the veranda to provide shelter for Ben on rainy days? Bookshelves? Yes…definitely bookshelves, even if he had nothing more than a few medical textbooks to put on them at the moment. When he thought about how welcoming Isla's house was, he could see the haphazard stacks of books, the overflowing baskets of wood for the log burner, the collections of seashells on the windowsill. He could almost smell the food being cooked in the kitchen, but…what he could *really* remember tasting was that kiss…

Jake blew out a breath and wound his thoughts back. He needed to scan the kitchen area of this store now and find pots and pans. And a fridge. That was a necessity that needed to be much higher on the list than any bookshelves. When his shift finished that day he had time to add some final items, including a television and a gaming console that made Arlo's eyes positively glow with excitement. The truck full of purchases arrived the next day and Jake and Arlo moved into their new home the day after that.

Ben came too.

And there they were.

Just the three of them. A man, boy and dog. Undeniably unconventional, but it felt like a family. When Jake checked that Arlo was okay and asleep, late that first night, and saw Ben lying on the end of the bed with his nose resting on Arlo's leg, he got a squeeze in his chest that made it hard to take a new breath. He knew what it was, even if the memory of feeling it was so faded.

It was love.

The bone-deep, unconditional kind of love that came from being part of the same family. If things had been different, it could have been like this for him and Troy. If only he'd been a bit older when they'd lost their mother so he could have provided a home for Troy and been mature enough to act in loco parentis. Jake couldn't turn back time, but what he could do was make up for having failed his baby brother.

So he renewed the promise he'd made the night Troy had died as he went down the wide central hallway of the old villa to his own bedroom. Nothing was going to be allowed to undermine that vow.

Arlo would come first from now on—for as long as he needed to be cared for.

No matter what.

It felt strangely quiet in the beach house.

The house felt empty.

Just the way Isla liked it. This was her favourite time of the day, where she could sit at the big old table and lose herself in the fantasy of the story she was creating. Even now, writing her tenth book, she could still feel the pull of letting that world close around her. Not forgetting the pain of reality, exactly, but being able to channel it into something different that had the ability to dilute it, at least temporarily.

It had probably saved her life in that first, unbearable year of having lost everything that mattered. Maybe it had even breathed life back into the part of her that could care. She'd created characters that she found she cared about and perhaps that had been enough to persuade her to go back, at least part-time, to the job that she'd once loved, of caring for people. A more distant kind of caring, mind you. Sometimes, Isla actually felt like one of the characters in her books as she threw herself into solving a medical mystery or using every skill she had in a dramatic fight to save a life. She'd learned to close the covers of that non-existent novel as she walked out of the hospital's doors at the end of a shift and that had helped, too. She had two things in her life that were related, one fictional and one real, but she had learned to channel and control her own emotional involvement in both the major components of what she'd been sure would be her entire life from now on.

But things were different now.

Isla found herself glancing away from her laptop screen, wondering where Ben was, forgetting for a heartbeat that she was no longer dog-sitting. Ben was apparently very happy as they all settled into the big house with its lovely garden and beautiful beach and forest walks within easy reach. There was no need for either Ben or Arlo to come and stay with Isla unless it was a weekend and Jake was working, but he was juggling his rosters with Sam and making that less likely. He'd also employed a high school student to be at home with Arlo after school and that might extend to weekends and overnights in the future so maybe Isla was being excused any significant involvement in their lives if that was her choice.

It might well have been her choice a few weeks ago.

But now it didn't feel right.

The house felt empty.

The pull of losing herself in a story that she really needed to finish was less inviting. She'd been staring at a blank screen for quite some time now and her brain was not cooperating. She did not need to add another sex scene to this book. What she did need to do was wind up the tension in a very different direction. She needed to set up the 'black moment' where it seemed that everything was ruined. Alex knew that Riley was onto him. If he was going to save himself, he was going to have to kill the woman he supposedly loved. She had it all worked out. Riley was going to find out the truth about what he'd done. And why. Alex was going to have to get rid of her in order to save himself. He had what he needed in the house. An ampoule of succinylcholine—the most commonly used paralytic agent for rapid sequence intubation. It had an onset of action of less than sixty seconds, would last long enough for the lack of ability to breathe to be fatal and, best of all, it was very hard to detect after death because of the rapid hydrolysis where water could break and disperse the chemical bonds. Riley would know exactly how terrifying it would be to die like that. This scene was going to be the biggest page-turner in the whole story.

Isla's fingers were poised over her keyboard. She started tapping.

'What made you want to be a doctor, Alex?' Riley needed to connect with Alex. To try and see if the man she'd fallen in love with had ever actually existed. 'To care for people? To save lives?'

'My twin brother died.' Alex's shrug made it seem that it should have been obvious. 'He got hit by a car on the way home from school and I was standing right beside him when it happened. The guy that was driving the car was only a few years older than us and he

was as high as a kite on drugs. I could see his face as he put his foot on the accelerator and drove away from the accident. Laughing...' The hatred in Alex's voice was chilling Riley to her bones. 'I'll never forget what he looked like, even if they'd never caught him. He's always there in my head. Always. Sometimes I see people that remind me of him—you know... The same dark hair. The age he would be now. They way they smile...'

Riley couldn't look away from him, despite the fear beginning to close in on her.

Dark hair, she thought. Like that young man that had that fatal asthma attack when he was under Alex's care. When she'd found the empty ampoule of an injectable beta blocker on the floor. And the one who'd come in with a dose of flu but had ended up dead at the foot of the stairs after that inexplicably aggressive incident. The kind of personality change that could happen if a blood sugar level crashed. If they'd had an overdose of insulin, perhaps—a drug that was very challenging to detect in a post-mortem.

They were all about the same age, those unexpected fatalities. Maybe Alex had wanted to learn to save lives when he'd been helpless as his twin brother died but there was poison there as well—a thirst for revenge for the person who'd been responsible.

Isla sighed. This scene didn't feel nearly exciting enough. What if she ramped up the stakes by having Alex moving in on Riley? Being confident and sexy? Scrambling her brain enough to make it hard for her to remember that she needed to be afraid of him. Very afraid…

With a frustrated growl, Isla gave up for the evening. She was *not* going to write another sex scene. Why was she even thinking about it?

Surely life would return to something closer to normal soon?

But she was thinking about Ben as she locked the front door with no need to go out onto the veranda again today. And Arlo as she walked past the spare room to get to the bathroom.

And, good grief… Why, oh, *why* couldn't she stop herself thinking about Jake Hammond as she stood in her shower a short time later, enjoying the slippery feeling of chasing soapsuds off her body with her hands?

'How's the house looking?' she asked Jake a few days later. 'Have you got everything you need? I've got far too much cutlery and too many coffee mugs if you need some.'

'Arlo and I had a ball choosing stuff in second-hand shops when we had a day in Auckland on the weekend. I even got a stack of old books, but the shelves still look too empty.'

Isla laughed. 'If it's just for decoration, I'll find some for you. My shelves could do with a good tidy-up.'

'That'd be great,' Jake said. 'I'll take a few of those Tessa Townsend ones. They're just what I need to unwind after a day in ED.'

Oh, help… The thought of Jake finding out who Tessa Townsend actually was made Isla feel suddenly shy enough to want to run and hide. Nobody knew that. Nobody really knew *her* anymore, did they? She didn't even know herself, really, because the person she *had* been no longer existed.

And that thought made her feel lonely. Which was odd because she'd spent years trying to shut herself away from people. To shut herself away from her memories.

'Bring them round after work one day,' Jake suggested casually, closing the patient notes he'd been scribbling an update into. 'You could see how well us boys are shaking down into the house. And we could cook for you.' His smile was one of those crinkly-eyed ones. 'We owe you a dinner or two.'

We…

Us boys. Jake, Arlo and Ben. An unusual but no less real family group.

That was making Isla feel as if she was missing out on something, but wasn't this exactly what she'd seen as the solution to an unwanted disruption to her life? She wasn't abandoning her sister's child but she didn't need to be risking something she wasn't capable of dealing with by becoming intimately involved.

'Or we could collect them,' Jake said. 'I need to talk to you later about this coming weekend. Sam's been covering for me a lot so I need to return the favour and let her go to a party in Auckland on Saturday night.' He looked up as Laura escorted a new patient into the department from the waiting room. 'I'll take this one,' he said. 'Maybe we can grab a walk if it gets quiet around lunchtime and I get a break. I like to pop back during the day if I can to check on Ben and it's your half day today, isn't it?' He raised an eyebrow. 'I think Ben's missing you,' he added casually. 'He'd like you to see his new kennel.'

Isla's first instinct was to refuse the invitation, but then she hesitated. It *was* her half day. There was no reason at all not to take a bit of time before she headed back to the east coast of the Coromandel peninsula.

She wanted to see Ben. The shock of knowing that Jake and Arlo were going to be living in a house that was so similar to her dream family home had worn off enough for curiosity to take its place. She wanted to see the inside of the old villa—the home that Jake was creating for her nephew.

So she found herself nodding slowly. 'Okay,' she agreed. 'If things are quiet enough for you to get away for a bit, I'd love to see Ben. And your house.'

Things were very quiet after midday, with one person on a cardiac monitor displaying a very normal heart rhythm despite the patient complaining that it had 'stopped' for long enough to make them faint earlier today. A baby running a slight temperature was also being watched to see if a dose of paracetamol was helping, mainly because the anxious mother needed support. Someone else needed stitches for a badly sliced finger—the sort of minor surgery that Sam was always keen to handle.

'I've got this,' she told them. 'Go and see that gorgeous dog of yours, Jake.'

There was nobody to blink an eye at two of Coromandel Hospital's doctors in their scrubs wandering over the helicopter landing pad in the early afternoon sunshine and going into the tree-lined street where Jake lived. Ben was so pleased to see Isla that his tail-wagging made his whole body wiggle with joy. It felt as if she was absorbing slivers of that appreciation of life as she rubbed his ears. She was still smiling as the dog followed them up the steps to the veranda and then through the front door into the wide hallway with its lovely polished wooden floor and a plaster archway halfway down.

They walked straight to the kitchen at the other end of the hallway, which still had an ancient coal-burning stove installed.

'Just for decoration,' Jake said. 'We've got all the mod cons we need as well.'

They worked their way back through the house for the tour.

The huge living area still had an ornate carved wooden fireplace around where a wood burner had been put in. Another room was set up as a study with an antique desk and a couple of bookshelves, empty apart from large medical textbooks filling a bottom shelf. The bathroom had a claw foot tub, brass taps and a mosaic tile floor.

'Arlo's room is already a mess.' Jake shook his head as he opened another door. 'I hate to think what it's going to be like when he hits his teens.'

Isla saw the dog bed in the corner of the room. 'Does Ben use that?'

Jake shook his head again. 'I look in on him every

night and they're cuddled up together on the bed. I'm cool with that. I'm pretty sure the benefits outweigh any disadvantages.' He shrugged and moved on. 'And that's about it. Just my room, here.'

Isla looked through the door.

'Also a bit messy.' Jake grimaced. 'Oops… I forgot I hadn't made my bed properly this morning. Haven't quite mastered the parental routine of getting a kid ready for school and making a lunch box and getting myself ready for work at the same time.'

Isla didn't want to think about all the things she was dodging when it came to Arlo's care and Jake's voice was just a background rumble as she briefly scanned the lovely bay window with its view to the garden and then the old fireplace with its register grate of pretty tiles. What wasn't brief was the way she was looking at the rumpled bedding and the dent in a pillow where Jake's head had clearly been during the night. She couldn't drag her gaze away from it, in fact. Where was the discarded sleepwear? Or did Jake sleep naked?

Oh, *my…*

A flicker had ignited deep in her body. Kind of like the one she'd had in the shower the other night that had made her feel so overheated she'd ended up turning the temperature of the water down to give herself a blast of icy rain to bring her back to reality before she got out.

There was no possibility of dousing herself with cold water right now. And Jake was standing so close to her in this doorway that she could feel the heat of his body adding what could have been rocket fuel to that flicker. When she finally shifted her gaze, she realised that she'd only made things worse. Instead of imagining a gorgeous naked man in that big bed, she was looking at Jake Hammond himself.

And he was looking straight back at her.

The electricity in the air was palpable. A fizzing sensation that filled the air between them and their thin cotton scrubs felt as if they were being vaporised by the heat being generated.

'We—' The word was so strangled that Isla had to clear her throat to make it coherent. 'I mean you... should probably be getting back to work.'

'Probably.' Jake's response was no more than a murmur. His gaze dropped from Isla's eyes to her lips. 'But Sam's more than capable and... I don't think I want to go anywhere else just yet.'

Isla could feel the world outside slipping into irrelevance. 'Me neither,' she whispered.

'What I want...' Jake said as he tilted and dipped his head very, very slowly, his gaze still locked on hers '...is to kiss you, Isla Preston.'

His head kept moving so that by the time he'd finished speaking, his lips were almost touching hers. She only needed to tilt her chin and they *would* be touching. *Kissing...*

There was no way in the world that Isla could talk herself out of making that movement. If she was honest, the thought of not kissing Jake didn't even occur to her.

Their lips touched softly for a heartbeat, and then something was unleashed that hadn't been there that first time this had happened. Something raw and fierce that made Isla part her lips and find Jake's tongue with her own. This was purely physical—a desperate need for this intimate human touch. To feel it—and taste it—with her whole body and not just her mouth. She wanted this. She wanted it more than she'd ever wanted anything in her life.

Jake must have sensed her need. Or maybe he felt it himself. Isla simply melted with the pleasure of feeling herself being pushed through the doorway into his bedroom with his lips still moving on hers. They broke apart just long enough for Isla to raise her arms and let Jake peel off the tunic of her scrubs and then the kiss reached a totally new level as she felt his hands on the bare skin of her back. She cried out softly with the shaft of sensation as his hands drifted over the thin layer of lace covering her breasts. She felt the edge of the bed behind her knees and fell backwards, cradled in Jake's arms. That broke the kiss enough for him to catch, and hold, her gaze.

'This is not a good idea,' he said softly.

'I know…'

'We should probably stop.'

'Mmm…' But Isla didn't look away.

'I don't want to,' Jake whispered. 'Do you?'

'No…' She ran her tongue over suddenly dry lips and heard a faint groan from Jake.

'Just once?'

'Yes…' This was perfect. She needed to do this just once. Just to see if it was possible to feel…this truly *alive* for just a little longer. 'But…'

'It's okay…' Jake leaned away to open the drawer of his bedside table. 'I'll keep you safe, Isla…'

CHAPTER NINE

ISLA DIDN'T REALLY need to go to Thames on any of her days off for the rest of that week but there was a garden centre that she hadn't visited for a while and when she texted Jake to tell him she'd collected a box of books that included some childhood classics Arlo might like, he'd invited her to dinner.

So, here she was, in the kitchen of the old villa, doing her best to focus on showing Arlo the books that she'd brought with him in mind and banish the thoughts of what had happened the first time she'd set foot in this house.

Thoughts that had been overwhelming anything else from the moment Jake had opened the front door for her and then caught her gaze as they walked past his bedroom door. She wasn't just thinking those thoughts either. She was feeling them, like an actual caress on her skin. She could almost *taste* them...

To be honest, they'd been there ever since she'd walked out of the house the day before yesterday but she had also been doing her best to relegate the memories of that extraordinary encounter to where it belonged. In the past already, because it couldn't happen again. Arlo had big enough adjustments in his life to get used to without what would be a confusing—and probably totally gross—development of his new aunt and uncle hooking up with each other.

Judging by how quickly Jake broke that eye contact, he was on exactly the same page. Arlo was in the house. They certainly weren't going to openly acknowledge what had happened between them. But it was there, in that heartbeat of eye contact.

It was there in the smile that Jake threw at Isla when she put the box of books on the kitchen table at one end of the big kitchen, as he went back to the bench and oven to finish making their dinner.

'These books might seem a bit old-fashioned,' Isla told Arlo. 'But they were stories I used to read to your mum and she loved them—even the ones I wasn't supposed to be reading to her, like the scary *Goosebumps* ones.'

'*You* read them to her?'

'I was a lot older than her and I loved reading aloud. She only wanted to listen when she was almost asleep, though. Or when it was raining too hard to be outside and she was bored, because what she really wanted to do was play on the beach. Or surf. I did, too. They used to say that those McGregor girls were born with seawater for blood.'

Arlo was staring at her, nodding slowly. He got that. Was the love of the ocean something that could be genetic? Not that it was enough of a connection to make her feel uncomfortably close to Arlo. It might still be in her blood but Isla hated the sea a lot more than she loved it these days.

'What are those books?' Arlo asked as she took out a boxed set.

'*The Chronicles of Narnia*. You might have heard of the first one—about the lion, the witch and the wardrobe?'

'I've seen the movie. It was really good.'

'Did you know that was filmed in New Zealand?'

Arlo's eyes widened. 'No way...'

Isla smiled at how impressed he was. 'One of the locations they used is a beach that's not far away from where I live. Cathedral Cove. It's my favourite beach ever. After Otara Bay, of course, because that's kind of mine.'

'Wow...can I go and see it?'

'Sure. I'll take you there some time when you come and stay for the weekend.'

'I'm coming this weekend, right?'

'Yes.' Isla was still smiling but what surprised her was the flash of anticipation that made it bigger. She was actually looking forward to having Arlo's company. She tried to push that emotion into the same mental space where she had just shoved everything X-rated. For the same reason, too. Emotions connected you to people and when you were connected you had something to lose.

Isla had no intention of letting connections like that get too big to be a threat. It was a relief to feel her personal distance growing as she let herself float away, into a safer space, on her next outward breath. Until Jake spoke and pulled her back into the moment.

'Hey...' Jake looked up from where he was standing by the kitchen bench. 'I'm working, remember? I want to go to Cathedral Cove too.'

'You're only working on Saturday, aren't you?' Arlo's eyebrows were hidden under his fringe as he turned back to Isla. 'Could we go on Sunday so Uncle Jake can come too?'

'Maybe,' Isla said. 'If the weather's good.'

Jake was checking his phone. 'Doesn't look great,' he said. 'But summer's almost here. I'm sure we could go soon.'

Arlo's attention had been diverted. 'You said I could go surfing again in summer. If I was better enough.'

'I did,' Jake agreed. 'And we've got that appointment coming up with the kidney specialist in Auckland next week. We'll see if he says it's okay.'

'The water will still be freezing,' Isla warned. 'It's not that warm, even in summer, if you're going to be in the water for a long time.'

'Probably still a lot warmer than Cornwall,' Jake suggested.

'We always used wetsuits,' Isla said.

'I *had* a wetsuit,' Arlo said. 'But it got left behind.' His face furrowed and Isla could almost feel him being pulled into the grief of everything he'd lost. His parents and friends, his home and beaches and the sport he loved. Her heart was breaking for him and she wanted to reach out and pull him into her arms. She wanted to reassure him that he still had people who cared about him. That there would be happy times ahead with endless beaches and waves to catch.

That things would get better. That the good things in life could make up for all the bad things that could happen.

She wasn't exactly the best person to convince him

of that but maybe Jake was. And maybe he knew why she couldn't do it, in the face of everything she'd lost, so that was why he had abandoned the potatoes he was peeling and was coming towards them.

'Hey…' His tone was gentle. 'We could go and get you a new wetsuit when we're in Auckland. How 'bout that?'

'Yeah…sure…' But Arlo was shrugging, as if it didn't really matter. He picked up one of the books. 'Can I go to my room?'

'Sure.' Jake's agreement echoed Arlo's. 'But dinner'll be ready in about twenty minutes, okay?'

Ben came out from under the table and followed Arlo out of the kitchen. They heard the door of his bedroom close a few seconds later.

Isla was alone in the kitchen with Jake. It would have been rude not to meet his gaze when she could feel him watching her put books back into the box.

'Thanks for these,' Jake said quietly. 'I think it's brilliant that you can give him something that was important to his mum.'

'Every house needs books,' Isla said. 'And if they're books that people have loved, it's part of what makes a house feel like a home.'

Jake's smile softened his whole face. 'Thanks for bringing them,' he said even more quietly. 'It's good to see you.'

Isla's mouth felt suddenly dry. It was way past time to break the eye contact they had but she couldn't do it. She wasn't even sure if her body was going to cooperate in staying upright. That electricity was there again, wasn't it? That fizzy air that made it hard to breathe.

She might be wearing jeans and a warm jumper this evening but it was no more protection than thin cotton scrubs had been against the heat that was being generated here.

Jake could feel it too. She could see it in his eyes. If Arlo hadn't been in his room just down the hallway and could pop back out at any moment, he'd be kissing her again right about now.

And, dammit, she'd be kissing him back.

Had they really thought that once would be enough?

Who had they been trying to kid?

It should be getting easier by now.

It had been nearly two weeks, for heaven's sake. More than enough time to have taken Arlo to the nephrology specialist in Auckland, to be given the all-clear for Arlo to do something as physical as surfing and to take him to a sportswear shop to purchase a wetsuit. The quiet joy he could see in Arlo's eyes as he came out of the changing cubicle, looking like a seal in the sleek black garment, gave Jake such a squeeze in his chest it prompted rather a lot more spending.

'Why don't we get you a new surfboard?' he suggested. 'That kids' size one Isla has must be more than twenty years old. Would it still be safe?'

The sales assistant who'd been helping Arlo find the right sized wetsuit shook his head. 'It would be too heavy,' he said. 'We have what we call softboards these days. Mix of foam and epoxy resin. Light enough for kids to carry themselves and buoyant enough to help keep them safe in the surf.'

Keeping Arlo safe sounded good to Jake. 'Let's take a look.'

The sales assistant grinned at Arlo. 'Wait till you see the one that looks like a slice of watermelon. It's too cool for school, mate.'

They loaded the bright red board with its black pips and the slice of green rind down one side into the car a short time later, along with the wetsuit and board wax and other necessities like a leg rope and fins. Jake's credit card had a large dent in it but it was worth it. Arlo might not be saying much but there was something new in how it felt to be together. Something closer that kept that squeezy feeling alive for Jake. This was the kind of thing he wished he could have done for Troy and it felt *so* good being able to do it for his brother's son.

There'd been enough time to drop Arlo off at Isla's house that weekend and pick him up, looking slightly sunburnt and smelling like the ocean, the next day. He didn't stop talking for the whole drive back to Thames.

'It's a cool beach. Isla says it's a lot calmer than Sailors Grave beach but I can only do it at high tide to start with and not in a big swell because there's rocks at each end. I had the beach all to myself, Uncle Jake! I've never been in the sea alone like that before.'

'Alone? You mean Isla wasn't there?'

'Oh, she was on the beach. She just didn't come into the water. She said she doesn't like getting wet these days.'

The squeeze on Jake's heart was not a happy one this time. How hard was it for Isla to even stand on a beach and look at the waves? Did she have nightmares about being in the sea after the accident that had claimed her entire family?

'Ben was there, too. He swam out at the end when he was sick of waiting for me to come in. I put him on top of my board and he stayed there while I took him back to shore. I think he really liked it.'

Isla gave the impression that she rather liked this new element in her relationship with her nephew. She talked to Jake about it when they arrived to work a shift together in Emergency a few days later.

'He's good,' she told Jake. 'The waves were small but he was up and riding them in no time. That surfboard is brilliant. Bright enough to be a spotlight on exactly where he is when you're watching him. He wants you to be there watching him next time.'

Working together had been all they'd done, of course. With them being the only two doctors on duty those days, there'd been no chance of taking a lunch break together. No chance of wandering around to his house for a bit of…

What *had* it been?

A bit of hanky-panky?

No. That was an insult to some mind-blowingly memorable sex.

It *had* been supposed to be a one-off. To get rid of that unexpected—and inappropriate—sexual tension that had sprouted from nowhere and exploded that day they'd been alone together in his new house.

Well…it had been an epic failure in that direction, hadn't it? If anything, it had made things worse. He wanted it to happen again, with a strength that was an unmissable red flag. Jake was well-practised in dealing with remnants of attraction that were still there after he'd ended a casual relationship before someone got hurt—i.e. the woman who wanted more from him than he was capable of giving—but, inexplicably, his tried and tested methods were proving ineffective this time.

The pull was, in fact, becoming more powerful.

Or was it simply feeling like this because Jake was currently driving towards Isla on a Sunday morning, after working a long shift yesterday that had made it too late to go and collect Arlo? A lovely sunny Sunday morning and he was about to spend the whole day in Isla and Arlo's company because this was the day they planned to go to Cathedral Cove.

Arlo had been torn between wanting to see the amazing beach that had been a movie location and not wanting to go because they'd have to leave Ben at home. He wasn't looking happy about Isla shutting the dog inside the house to stop him trying to follow them.

'But why can't we take him?'

'We've talked about this, Arlo. Dogs are not allowed on Cathedral Cove beach. It's a marine reserve and the Department of Conservation protects it. Dogs can be a threat to nesting birds or fragile ecosystems. It would be too hot to leave him in the car while we walk down to the cove. He'll be fine here for a few hours. You can take him for a run down at our beach when we get back, okay?'

'Okay,' Arlo muttered.

Our beach, Jake thought. Where a young boy could have the sea all to himself with just one woman there to watch. It seemed like a lonely image. Next time, he wanted to be there as well.

Minutes later, they were all in Jake's SUV for the half-hour drive north up the coastline to where they'd either need to get boat access to Cathedral Cove from the township of Hahei or do a forty-five minute walk from the start of the track at the top of the hill.

Jake would prefer to do the walk. That way, he could use the exercise and fresh air to help distract him from being so close to Isla. He might be more successful in banishing the errant thoughts that, rather than going on what felt like a family outing, he would prefer to be spending some time alone with her.

Alone.

And naked.

How many years had it been since Isla had gone to Cathedral Cove?

Too many?

Or not enough?

This outing had seemed like a good idea when she'd told Arlo about this beach being used for a movie and he'd been so keen to come and see it for himself. She'd been ready to get out of the house herself this weekend. She'd finished the manuscript of her latest Tessa Townsend medical thriller this week and she'd printed it out, ready for a final read-through and tweak before she sent it off to her editor. A couple of days' break would allow her to spot any glitches in the timeline or flow far more clearly.

But now that they were walking down the track,

Isla was starting to wonder whether she had underestimated the possible impact this could have. Memories were crowding in on her. The excitement of heading down the track with Sage, their parents behind them carrying all the paraphernalia they considered necessary for a proper picnic. It was a long walk with lots of steps. The last section that took them down the volcanic cliff face to the beach had dozens of wooden steps that were almost as steep as a ladder. It meant a breath-stealing climb back up at the end of the day for tired kids with sandy feet and sun-kissed skin but it was always worth it.

The two curved beaches, with their soft, blindingly white sand were separated by the enormous white stone archway and natural tunnel that had made this cove famous. The Pōhutukawa trees at the base of the cliffs provided shade but were not yet covered with their distinctive bright red flowers for summer, but it was just as gorgeous as she had always remembered it with the glints of sunshine on impossibly blue water as it crested and then foamed onto the shore in gentle waves.

'No good for surfing,' Arlo said.

'It is sometimes. Your mum and I always liked it like this, though. We came to swim and sunbathe and climb along the bottom of the cliffs and run through the tunnel and eat sandy sandwiches.'

'Yuck.' But Arlo couldn't hide a cheeky smile as he caught Isla's gaze and...*oh*...how had she not realised how much he looked like her baby sister?

She had to turn away to hide the sudden ache in her heart that might have shown on her face and dampened what was supposed to be a fun outing. Isla spread the blanket they'd brought with them under a Pōhutukawa tree and watched as Jake and Arlo wandered off to touch the smooth walls of the cliffs, admire the archway and walk through the tunnel to see the other half of the cove. She could see Jake using his phone to take photos. They were both looking awestruck when they returned.

'This goes to the top of my list of the world's most beautiful beaches,' Jake said.

Arlo was shading his eyes from the sun to look out to sea. A flotilla of kayaks came around the headland and slowed to take in the view of the cove.

'It's got an island,' Arlo said. 'Like our beach.'

'This one's got a name,' Isla told him. 'It's called the Smiling Sphinx Rock because it looks like the Egyptian statue at the pyramids. Have you seen that?'

Arlo shook his head.

Jake was tapping his phone screen. 'Come and look at this,' he invited Arlo, who went to sit beside him on the blanket.

'Yeah…it does kind of look like that.'

'See that flat rock that's closer to shore?'

Arlo nodded.

'I got into big trouble one day because I'd helped your mum swim out to it and she jumped off.'

'Why did you get into trouble?'

'Because I was supposed to be looking after her and you have to be very careful about how and when you jump off that rock. It was safe enough because it was nearly high tide and the waves were as flat as the rock, but our dad wasn't happy.' Isla shook her head as she caught Jake's glance. 'Sage was the fearless one. Always after an adventure.'

Jake was smiling. 'I suspect you were very alike. I totally get why my brother fell for her.'

Isla blinked. What did *that* mean?

Did Jake find her attractive? In more than a purely physical sense?

'I'm thirsty,' Arlo said. 'Can I have a drink, please?'

'Of course.' It was a relief to turn away from Jake and the rather disturbing direction her thoughts were trying to take her in. She pulled a can of soft drink from the picnic bag and handed it to Arlo. Then she took out the soft rolls she had made this morning, filled with shredded chicken and avocado and bacon left over from breakfast. She gave both Jake and Arlo one of the wrapped sandwiches and took one herself. The walk and the sea air had made her hungry and they couldn't stay here too long when they'd left Ben shut up in the house.

The kayakers vanished from sight behind the archway as they were eating their lunch but a yacht sailed into view and Isla suddenly found she wasn't hungry any longer.

Jake noticed her abandoning her food. Or maybe it was the way she was staring at the yacht.

'You okay?' he asked quietly. Then he followed her line of sight. '*Oh...*' was all he said.

Arlo looked from Jake to Isla and then to what they were now both staring at. 'What's wrong with that boat?' he asked. He looked back at Isla and his eyes narrowed as he frowned. 'You look…sad.' His tone was almost accusing.

Isla found herself nodding. 'I kind of am,' she told Arlo. 'I used to have a boat just like that. Or rather, *we* did. My husband Luke and our little boy, Max. And our dog, Ollie.' Her voice cracked. How long had it been since she'd said these names out loud? Brought them into her present instead of being hidden in her past?

Arlo was still frowning. 'Where are they?' He sounded puzzled now. 'Why do you live by yourself?'

'There was a horrible accident,' Isla said, her voice a whisper. 'We were all on our boat and we hit something in the middle of the night and…' she closed her eyes and swallowed hard '…and it tipped upside down into a big sea and…and I was the only one who survived.'

'How old was Max?' Arlo asked.

'Three. Nearly four.'

'What sort of dog was Ollie? Was he a border collie, like Ben?'

'No. He was a golden labrador. And he was a bit fat.' Isla tried to smile but it wasn't happening.

To her horror, Isla could feel the prickle of tears forming. She hadn't cried for years. Not since she'd finally found a form of peace in being able to step back from getting too emotionally involved in anything. About the same time she'd found she could channel that emotion into fiction and still keep herself safe.

She didn't feel safe right now.

'Hey…' Jake got to his feet. 'Come with me, Arlo. I want to get a photo of you with the sphinx rock behind you.'

'But—'

Whatever it was in Jake's tone or the look he gave Arlo was enough to have them both walking away a moment later. Isla could see that Jake was talking to Arlo by the way his head was bent. Was he explaining that she needed a moment to herself? Or that perhaps she didn't want to say anything more about her past?

Maybe he was talking to Arlo about his own loss. About the connection they all had and why it was so lucky they'd found each other because they were the people who could really understand. And care…

The threat of tears evaporated for Isla. But something just as disturbing was taking their place.

That feeling of caring. A mix of whatever it had been that had prompted her to tell Arlo part of her own story, seeing the likeness to her sister in his face and…that comment Jake had made about getting why Troy had fallen for Sage. And why on earth hadn't she realised that this would end up feeling like a family outing, which was probably why she had been drawn back into the past so far. Past more than one of those carefully constructed protective barriers.

Had they been breached? Beyond repair?

This was…scary.

Terrifying, even.

But not because she was finding herself in a space she'd been so sure she never wanted to enter again.

It was because she was starting to think it might be *exactly* what she wanted.

CHAPTER TEN

IT SEEMED TO take far longer to walk back up the hill to the parking area than it had to head towards the beach that had proved just as stunning as Jake had been led to believe

The effort of getting up the steepest sections was enough to keep them all out of breath and stop them trying to make conversation. Arlo led the way and Jake suspected that was because he was worried about Ben being shut in Isla's house. At least when Arlo was at school in Thames, Ben had the run of the garden. The bond between this dog and boy was pure gold as far as Jake was concerned. Ben had done far more than either he or Isla could have achieved in the way of providing comfort, companionship and an anchor that he could use to settle into a totally new life.

Jake was bringing up the rear as they climbed more slowly on the longest uphill stretch. He wasn't thinking about Arlo right now. He was watching the long, dark braid of Isla's hair swinging against her back a few steps in front of him and thinking about what she'd told Arlo. She'd given him only the barest bones of her tragic story but Jake could see the whole shape of it all too clearly.

They'd been a family. She'd loved her husband and adored their son and they'd had a dog—overweight not just because he was a labrador but because they'd all loved him and probably gave him too many treats. They'd been her family. Her world, and…dear Lord, his heart had broken right along with her voice when she had been telling Arlo their names. He'd wanted so much to wrap his arms around her. To tell her that he understood why she'd needed to protect herself so fiercely from getting too close to anyone else.

That he was proud of her for not turning her back on Arlo and even more so for showing a glimpse of who she really was—or had been. She was making herself very vulnerable and Jake was well aware of how easily she could be frightened and disappear behind those barriers again. That was why, instead of saying anything to Isla, he'd taken Arlo for a quiet word out of earshot.

Maybe it was too much to ask of a nine-year-old but Arlo had had to take on a lot of what being an adult was all about when his life had changed so dramatically. He, of all people, was the one who could understand what Isla had gone through and she might be the only person in his world who really understood the magnitude of what he had lost himself. So, Jake was banking on Arlo caring enough about Isla to not want to risk making her vanish from their lives.

Jake certainly didn't want Isla to vanish. Quite the opposite.

Isla pointed out a side road on the way home that she said led to Hot Water Beach.

'A beach…with *hot* water?' Arlo shook his head. 'I don't believe you.'

'It's true,' Isla insisted. 'There are geothermal springs beneath the sand and if you know the right spots you can see them bubbling up around low tide. It's a really popular thing for tourists to go there and dig holes and sit in the hot water. We can go there one day.'

'Okay.' But Arlo didn't sound particularly interested. He just wanted to get back to the beach house, and as soon as they arrived he asked if he could take Ben for a walk on the beach.

'Sure,' Isla said. 'Give me five minutes to have a shower and get changed. I'm still hot and sticky after walking up the Cathedral Cove hill. Unless you want Uncle Jake to go with you?'

'No… I want to take Ben by myself,' Arlo said. 'You said you and Mum were allowed to be on the beach by yourselves.'

'That's true.' Isla nodded. 'But there were rules. We weren't allowed to go out on the rocks or get wet. Not even paddling.'

Arlo shrugged. 'I just want to throw sticks for Ben. And maybe see if the teepee is still there.'

'If it's okay with your Uncle Jake, it's okay with me,' Isla said.

She caught Jake's gaze and this felt as if they were making a joint decision. Co-parenting. He liked that.

'You get the same rules that your mum had,' he told Arlo. 'Take your phone so you can call if you need to. And don't be more than an hour or we'll come looking for you. We'll need to head home then.'

He watched Arlo and Ben disappear through the door and then turned to Isla. 'Why don't you have that shower? I'll have a cup of tea ready for when you get out. Or coffee?'

'Tea would be perfect. And I will go and jump in the shower. I can still feel sand in my shoes. And possibly in other places.'

Jake tried very hard not to imagine any other places on Isla's body where any sand might be lingering. As the kettle boiled, he distracted himself by wandering around the living area. He paused by a pile of paper beside a closed laptop. Two piles. One face down, as if someone was halfway through the process of reading the pages. Without realising what he was doing, Jake found himself beginning to read the top page of the face-up pile. And then he blinked and turned over the face-down pile to find the title page of what was, quite clearly, the manuscript of a novel.

Code... Revenge was in bold letters. At the bottom of the page in smaller letters was—*by Tessa Townsend*.

Jake's jaw dropped. *Isla* was Tessa Townsend?

Of course she was. It explained why she had copies of every one of this author's books on her shelves, yet she'd dismissed her as being an 'okay' rather than brilliant writer. It was another secret that gave him even more insight into the real Isla. A bond that felt as if it was pulling them even more closely together.

With this knowledge, Jake couldn't help himself. He went back to the page he'd started reading.

...how could she start talking about work and these

fatal cases that were increasingly bothering her when he was giving her 'the look'?...

Jake read faster. It felt as if the words were scorching his eyeballs.

...She always closed her eyes, waiting for the moment his finger would touch her lips, because she knew what was coming next. His lips, on top of hers, his hands cradling her head now—kissing her so thoroughly her bones were melting and he would have to scoop her up into his arms and carry her to their bed and...

Oh, *man*…

Jake was so engrossed in what he was reading that he didn't realise Isla had come into the room until he heard her horrified gasp.

'What are you *doing*?' Her voice was shocked. 'That's *private*!'

He should apologise for snooping. Reassure her that her secret was safe with him. He could say that he was more than impressed to find out what she did when she wasn't engaged in her other life as an emergency specialist. But Jake said none of those things. He stayed silent as he walked towards where Isla was standing outside the bathroom door. He could feel the warmth of the steamy air escaping the room as he got close enough. Isla's gaze was fixed on his, her lips slightly parted. He could feel the warmth of her body as he put the pad of his finger against the middle of her forehead. Still without saying a word, without even the hint of a smile, holding that eye contact, he traced the outline of her face until his finger found the softness of those parted lips and then he let his fingers thread themselves gently into her hair as she tilted her face to meet his lips with her own.

Was this kiss melting her bones?

It was certainly melting Jake's. He was lost in it.

Or maybe it wasn't just this kiss he was lost in.

This felt like a whole new world. He was in a space he'd never been in before. A space that was limitless and beyond beautiful and where everybody wanted to get to but it was also a forbidden space because Jake knew he didn't have a passport. He hadn't qualified to be allowed entry. This was where people went when they loved someone enough to be able to protect them and care for them for as long as you could draw breath, and he'd failed miserably the last time he'd been here. His expulsion might have been voluntary, and he was actually trying to reverse that decision but...had he earned the right to be here?

To be in love with Isla?

An odd clicking became faintly audible and it almost sounded like someone tutting their disapproval but then the bang of a door broke the moment—and this astonishing kiss—with an unpleasantly sharp jolt. Jake looked up to see Ben walking into the room, his nails tapping on the bare wooden boards. The front door behind the dog was swinging and banged again as it failed to latch.

That door had been closed a moment ago and Ben couldn't have opened it.

'Arlo?'

There was no response to Jake's call and realisation hit with enough force to make him groan.

'Oh, *no…*'

'He saw us,' Isla whispered. 'Didn't he?'

'I'm guessing so.' Jake pressed his palm to his forehead. 'I'd better go and talk to him.'

'Want me to come too?'

'No.' Jake shook his head, heading towards the door with Ben at his heels. This was one thing he was sure of. 'Best I do this alone.'

Isla went into the kitchen and made a pot of tea. She heard a car door slam and then there was silence outside.

What would Arlo be thinking? How shocked would he have been to see his mother's sister and his father's brother *kissing* each other like that? It had to be confusing enough to feel like some kind of betrayal and that was the last thing this child needed, just when he was starting to feel grounded in his new life. How could it not have occurred to them that he could come back from the beach at any moment?

She couldn't blame it all on Jake, even if he had invaded her privacy and read part of her manuscript. That he'd acted out what he'd been reading with such intensity was possibly the best compliment her writing had ever been given. She couldn't deny that she'd been thinking about him when she'd written it in the first place. Or that it had been even better in reality.

So good.

A kiss like none she'd ever had before. Because this

one was reminding her of *everything* she'd ever had before.

And everything she'd ever lost…

How had she allowed this to happen? The only reason she had let Jake slip past her defences had been because Arlo had provided a connection. A bridge? It wasn't that she'd been so determined not to let her nephew close enough to capture her heart, it was because she'd believed that she wasn't capable of feeling that kind of love again. Ever. Not for a child—especially a *boy*—even if she shared a genetic bond with him.

Did this mean that she *was* still capable of those feelings? Emotional connection that was entirely different to the purely physical attraction she'd been unable to resist when it came to Jake?

The remorse she was feeling right now suggested that might be true. Isla felt terrible that Arlo might be distressed by what he'd walked in on. Her heart was actually aching so much that Isla pressed her hand to her chest.

She didn't want to feel like this. She didn't want these feelings. She never wanted to love anybody so much that it would feel like the end of the world if she lost them. She turned swiftly as the front door opened and that ache in her heart went up several notches as she saw the expression on Jake's face

She was in trouble here. Was it even possible to back off and pull up the drawbridge? To get back inside that emotional fortress she'd built to keep her heart—and herself—safe?

* * *

'We're going to head home,' Jake said.

Isla pulled in a breath. 'Is he upset?'

'He said he's really tired and that's why he didn't stay long at the beach. But yes… I think he's upset. He won't say he saw anything but I think he's just protecting himself from something he might see as a threat.'

Jake could see the way Isla's eyes darkened.

She caught her bottom lip between her teeth and he could imagine how hard she was biting it. Of all people, Isla could understand the kind of threat that trusting people—*loving* them—could bring, but Jake knew he had to be very clear about this.

Because this was his fault.

'If he thinks we're hooking up,' he added quietly, 'he might feel as if he's in the way. That he's not wanted. That there isn't a single person in the world that really wants him.'

They stared at each other. The only reason they'd become as close as they had was because of Arlo. Because they'd been putting this child's needs ahead of their own. This could have undone any progress they'd made and they were risking never being able to repair the damage. Jake was facing failure in his ability to protect and care for another human.

'I told him it meant nothing,' Jake said. 'And that it won't happen again.'

It had never been meant to happen in the first place.

It had simply been irresistible.

Selfish.

'I told him that we were friends,' Jake added. 'And

that we intended to co-parent him for as long as he needs us. That's true, isn't it?'

Isla was nodding but she wasn't making eye contact.

'Neither of us want anything more than that. We both knew that, didn't we?'

'Yes.' The response was no more than a whisper. She still wasn't looking at him but then she spoke more decisively. 'Absolutely.'

It *was* true. They'd both been completely honest about their determination not to get involved in anything like a relationship. They'd made a joke about not wanting that first kiss to make it seem as if they'd been hitting on each other. Jake had confessed his 'love 'em and leave 'em' reputation. Isla had told him that she was never going to try and replace what she had lost because she knew it was totally impossible.

An unexpected attraction had simply gone too far.

Far enough for Isla to tell Jake that she wasn't going to walk away from Arlo because he was the only family she was ever going to have. He felt that same responsibility—maybe even more so because this was Troy's child and he had, in effect, walked away from his younger brother. Neither of them had walked away from Arlo but they'd done something that might have pushed *him* away.

Isla finally looked up and caught his gaze. 'We need to fix this,' she said quietly. 'What can I do?'

'Just lay low for a bit,' Jake suggested. 'I'll take him home. Maybe I'll tell him about you being a writer and me reading about that kiss in your new story and it was just a bit of silliness. He doesn't need to know anything else.'

A bit of silliness. Anything else that had happened between them was also being dismissed.

Isla took a deep breath. 'That's fine by me. I'm certainly not going to say anything. To anyone.'

'See you at work?'

'In a couple of days. I've taken a bit of time this week so I can meet my publishing deadline. I've still got a lot of proofreading and editing to do.'

It felt too hard to take in a new breath because Jake's chest was suddenly full of something other than air but it took a moment to pick out which emotion had the biggest percentage of space. Was it regret—that he could never kiss Isla again, let alone make love to her? Or shame, that he'd let it happen in the first place? Okay… the concern for Arlo definitely trumped either of those feelings but there was something else there as well. Something unexpected. Pride, in Isla's secret talent?

'It's going to be a great book,' he said softly. 'I can't wait to read the rest of it.'

To Isla's surprise, Jake wasn't at work when she arrived at Coromandel Hospital for her first shift that week.

'Apparently Arlo's not well enough to go to school,' Sam Gillespie told her. 'So I'm covering for Jake.'

Isla called Jake as soon as she got some free time between patients. 'I heard about Arlo,' she said. 'How sick is he?'

'I'm not sure,' Jake said. She could hear his footsteps on the wooden floor of his house and then a door closing. Was he walking into the garden to be out of Arlo's earshot? 'He's tired and not eating much and he's running a bit of a temperature. Nothing alarming and he might just be coming down with a cold or something but I want to keep an eye on him today and see how much he's peeing.'

'Do you think it's a kidney problem?' The stab of concern was sharper than anything Isla normally felt for any patient, even children and babies.

'Maybe he's pushed things a bit hard with the surfing or something. I don't want to take any chances. Not when he's only got one kidney and that's been damaged recently.'

'Want me to drop some dipsticks around? Nice easy way to check protein or blood in the urine.'

'I would like to do a blood test. Get creatinine and electrolyte levels.'

'Bring him in. We could do that today.'

'I should take him to the local medical centre. Do you know any of the GPs enough to recommend someone?'

'Yes. I'd go to Adam Carter. He's really good, especially with kids. He's got a little girl himself, Charlotte. He always follows up his patients who end up being admitted or seen in the emergency department here and I know he's very diligent. If he knows Arlo's seeing a specialist in Auckland he'll take this seriously.'

She heard Jake's sigh.

'Are you okay?' she asked quietly. 'Is Arlo still upset about…you know…?'

'I'm fine,' Jake said. 'Just a bit worried. I'll see if I

can get an appointment with Adam Carter. And no, I don't think he's upset any longer. Just not very well.'

'Let me know if there's anything I can do.' Isla glanced up at the clock on the staffroom wall. It was time she headed back into the department. She was about to end the call when Jake spoke again.

'There is something,' he said.

'What?'

'We haven't talked about it, but now might be a good time to think about it, at least.'

'Oh...?' Isla knew where this was heading but she wasn't quite ready to put it into words.

'I told you that I'm out of the picture as a donor if Arlo ever needs a kidney.'

There was a moment's silence. It was Isla who broke it.

'And I'm the only other family he's got,' she said quietly. 'So I should get tested.'

'No pressure,' Jake said.

Isla wasn't feeling pressured. What she *was* feeling was relieved. This was something she could do for Arlo that didn't require a risky level of emotional involvement. She wasn't exactly being the model aunt of an orphaned child. Maybe this could go some way to making up for that.

'It's a no-brainer,' she told Jake. 'I should have already done it. I'll look into what tests are required today. And, Jake...?'

'Yes?'

'Keep me posted.'

As much as she was trying to put a lid on how concerned she was feeling, it was impossible not to care. But that was okay, wasn't it? She cared about all her patients. She had learned to make sure that there was enough of a buffer zone to keep it completely separate from her private life. She needed to think of Arlo as a patient for the duration of his illness. To take any emotional reaction out of the equation by focusing on clinical details.

It almost worked.

Until Jake phoned her that afternoon.

'Adam's concerned,' he said succinctly. 'He's got flank pain and his temperature's over thirty-nine degrees Celsius now. Given his history of serious kidney injury and the fact that he's only got one kidney, that puts him at high risk for acute pyelonephritis. He got straight onto the renal specialists in Auckland and Arlo's going to be admitted for tests, including an urgent CT scan. He may need IV antibiotics for a few days.'

Isla did her best to focus on the clinical details. 'Could this be related to the injury?'

'That's a possibility. Scarring on a kidney can disrupt urine flow and inflammation of kidney tissue can weaken immunity for quite some time. We'll know more later. I'd better get back inside. I've left Arlo collecting things like his tablet and some books but we need to hit the road asap.'

'What can I do to help?'

'Could you stay at our place tonight and look after Ben?'

'Yes, of course.'

'Are you on duty tomorrow?'

'Yes.'

There was a short silence. 'Could you have a chat with Polly and see if they can find cover for you?'

'Why?'

Something squeezed Isla's heart hard enough to make her catch her breath. Did Jake need her by his side in what could become another crisis?

Did *Arlo* need her?

'If this does turn out to be serious, we might have to fast-track finding out whether you're a match. If you can get up to Auckland for a few hours and meet the transplant team, you could get most of the testing process underway.'

Isla found herself letting her breath out in a sigh. That squeeze had turned into an ache and she knew it held an element of hurt but she pushed it aside. Hard. This was good.

Clinical.

Better than simply clinical details though. Going through the process of testing, and possibly becoming, an organ donor for her nephew would surely go a long way to balancing any guilt for increasing the emotional distance between them enough to provide protection.

It wasn't just for herself. Jake wanted this as well.

It was better for all of them.

CHAPTER ELEVEN

THE YOUNG DOCTOR from the renal transplant team, Indira, welcomed Isla to her initial interview.

'Thank you so much for making yourself available so promptly. I understand you're Arlo's aunt?'

'Yes. His mother Sage was my younger sister.'

Isla had driven up to Auckland early this morning. Sam was going to check on Ben during the day and would stay over at Jake's house if, for some reason, she couldn't get back to Thames this afternoon.

Arlo's kidney infection had been confirmed within hours of his arrival in Auckland Children's Hospital yesterday. He had been admitted to the renal ward, was going to be on IV antibiotics for at least forty-eight hours and he was being closely monitored for any signs that the infection could be causing irreversible damage to his solitary kidney.

'Perfect,' Indira said. 'And you're a doctor yourself, like his Uncle Jake?'

'I am.'

Indira was sorting a rather thick pile of forms in front of her. 'What an astonishing coincidence that you were working together without knowing the connection you had.'

'Yes.'

Isla could feel how tight her smile was. She didn't want to discuss that connection. It would be preferable to not even think about it.

There was no need for anybody else to know how that connection had blown out of control. It was over now and there had been a good reason that it had happened in the first place. She'd been alone for a long time. The need for both companionship and physical touch had been bottled up, unwanted and ignored for long enough to need attention. Allowing herself to acknowledge the attraction to Jake had been release of pressure, that was all. And it had been dealt with. Fortunately, Jake felt the same way she did about staying clear of significant relationships. They could easily wind this back to what *could* last without the risk of even more disruption to their lives. Or Arlo's.

They could be friends. That would take care of any need for companionship for Isla. Controlled companionship in manageable bites of time.

And sex?

Well, who knew? Maybe, in the future, it could turn into a friendship with benefits. Way in the future. When Arlo wasn't so vulnerable. If Jake was still single.

It wasn't as if she was ever going to find that kind of connection with anyone else. She hadn't consciously missed it before his presence in her life became anything more than being a colleague. She might be feeling the absence of it in the wake of the agreement that it had to stop but that would fade soon enough.

Wouldn't it?

Distance, she reminded herself. That was the key.

Indira had finished arranging the paperwork. Isla could see laboratory test requests and what looked like information sheets and consent forms. 'Are you familiar with the testing process for organ donation?'

'Only in general terms. I certainly didn't expect to be involved personally.'

'But you're happy to proceed?'

'Yes. Of course.' She managed to hold the searching gaze she was under. 'Arlo's my nephew.'

'That doesn't mean you have to go through with this because of the expectations of others—or what you perceive as your duty,' Indira said. 'It's part of our responsibility to your welfare to make sure you're not being coerced or that it might result in stress that would be a risk to your own mental health. I've got you scheduled for a chat with our psychologist later this morning, if that's okay?'

Isla nodded this time but she couldn't smile. She was going to have to talk about her past, wasn't she? About the horror of losing her entire family and the depression that had been such a struggle to overcome. Could she do that and be convincing in claiming that she was coping well these days? Well enough to cope with her involvement with Arlo and potential major surgery for him and herself?

'We'll get on with the first tests before that,' Indira continued. 'Some blood tests to cover all the usual health checks like kidney and liver functions, HIV and hepatitis et cetera. It'll just be some extra blood for the blood typing and cross-match testing. We'll also do a physical exam, a twelve-lead ECG to check on your heart function and take some chest X-rays. Any questions so far?'

Isla managed another smile this time. 'Sounds like a good warrant of fitness to be getting. How long will it all take?'

'A lot of the results will be available fast—today, even—and we would, of course, stop the process at any time if something concerning shows up.'

Like the stress factors her past presented? Or did Arlo have antibodies that would attack her tissue and she'd fail the cross-match tests like Jake had? What would happen then? How sick would Arlo *get*? Could it be fatal? Isla swallowed hard and took a mental step back. A big step.

Perhaps Indira had sensed what she'd been thinking about.

'The tissue typing needs samples from both you and Arlo and involves more specialised lab work so it could take several days. Maybe a week.' But she was smiling. 'Or did you mean how long would it take for you to jump through all the hoops today? Don't worry, I expect you'll still be able to visit Arlo and get home in time for dinner. It's possible that Arlo could be discharged today even and go home on oral therapy. He's feeling a lot better.'

'That's good to hear.'

So good, Isla could feel a lump forming in her throat. Oh, help…she never got lumps in her throat when she knew her patients were on the road to recovery earlier and more easily than expected. She needed to work harder on being professional.

Distant.

She cleared her throat, hoping that would make the lump disintegrate. She also pasted a brighter smile onto her face.

'What's first?' she asked. 'Bloods? I did send some through to the labs yesterday for a complete blood count and kidney and liver function. Those results might be available by now, which might speed things up?'

'Indeed.' Indira nodded. 'I can do the ECG and a quick physical here.' She picked up an arm cuff. 'Let's get this process underway by seeing what your blood pressure is.'

'I've passed everything so far,' Isla said. 'My blood pressure's normal, my heart's in good shape and there's nothing wrong with my lungs. Even the psychologist thought I was normal.' She was smiling at Jake. 'I didn't tell her I write down my fantasies of murdering people, mind you.'

Jake laughed. He'd arranged to meet Isla in the hospital café for a very late lunch when she'd texted him a short time ago to say she'd finished all the testing.

'I'm sure she'd be as impressed as I was to find out that you're Tessa Townsend,' he said.

'*Shh…*' Isla made an agonised face. 'That's our secret, remember?'

'As if I'd ever forget.' Jake's smile faded. 'I won't forget this either, Isla.'

'What? This lunch?' Isla looked down at her half-eaten muffin. 'I thought it was a bit dry, to be honest.'

'You know what I mean. You doing this. Being tested. Being prepared to go through with a kidney donation if it's needed.'

Isla looked away. Being looked at like she was so special made it very difficult to keep that essential distance.

'It's the least I can do, really,' she said, her shoulders lifting in a small shrug. 'It's not just for Arlo. Or even for Sage. It would make me feel better about who I am and how I've chosen to live my life.'

Jake wanted her to look back at him. To meet his gaze so that he could try and communicate that he understood exactly what she wasn't saying. That a kidney was a much easier part of her body to give away than any part of her heart. Of course he understood. He felt the same way. He'd spent the whole of his adult life being resolute in not giving away his heart. Because he knew it wasn't a good enough gift.

That he'd failed Troy. His kid brother. The person he'd loved the most.

He'd come too close to failing Arlo as well, but it felt as if they were getting past the hiccup of him being caught kissing Isla. Having sworn Arlo to secrecy, he'd told him about Isla's hidden life as a writer and how reading that kiss in her book had given him the crazy idea of trying it out. Perhaps there'd been enough of the truth in his cover-up to make it plausible. Or maybe Arlo thought that accepting his excuse and promises that it would never happen again or interfere with their lives together was the quickest way out of a conversation he'd prefer not to be having.

The way Isla was avoiding eye contact made it seem like she was looking for an escape from this conversation.

'Let's hope it's never needed,' he said. 'Arlo's looking so much better I think they're going to let me take him home later today.'

Isla was smiling now, a smile that reached her eyes, and Jake couldn't look away. He'd known she had beautiful eyes but he'd thought of them as being simply brown, like his. A perfect match for her dark hair. How had he not noticed that they could light up with an almost golden glow that made them a dark hazel rather than brown. Burnt caramel, that was what they looked like.

They were, in fact, the most beautiful eyes he'd ever seen. Ever. He could have sat there for a long time, simply looking into them, but he forced himself to look away. Friends—or co-parents—did not stare into each other's eyes like star-crossed lovers making their final farewells.

'I might have a hard job persuading Arlo to get out of bed and get dressed,' he said lightly. 'He won't take his nose out of his books. He's on the third one of the Narnia series now and he's totally into it.'

'That was one of my childhood faves.' Isla nodded. 'I kept all those books because I was so much looking forward to reading them to Max one day.' She closed her eyes and blew out a breath as if she was dismissing that peek into a past that was still too painful to visit. 'I love that Arlo's into reading. I've always believed that the joy, or even just escape, that books can bring is one of the only kinds of real magic in the world.'

'Is writing them even better than reading them?'

Oh…that thoughtful look on Isla's face made Jake want to smile again. No…if he was honest, it made him want to trace the shape of her whole face with his fingertips again. Until he got to her mouth and then he'd slide them into her hair and—

'No.'

The word was firm enough to sound like a reprimand for where his thoughts were going. Quite right, too. Friends didn't fantasise about kissing each other.

'It's too intense,' Isla said. 'And you have to keep part of your brain distant enough to be aware of the bigger picture—of how the whole story's fitting together or what's happening with your character's emotional arc. You can't just fall into it and get swept away like you can when you're reading. Or listening. I like how long it takes me to drive to work these days because I can listen to people reading me stories and that's like remembering Mum or Dad reading to me at bedtime.' Her eyes were still shining. 'It's like…a hug.'

She glanced at her watch. 'I should get going,' she said. 'I can take Ben for a walk when I get back. Let me know if you'll be bringing Arlo home later and I'll make some dinner. We'll need to talk about looking after Arlo for however long he needs to be off school.'

Jake watched her walk out of the café.

He drew in a deep, slow breath. This was how it needed to be. If there was one thing he needed to do better than anything else in his life so far, it was to be a parent to Arlo. To make up for every failure he'd ever made with anyone else he'd cared about. He had come too close to messing up this opportunity to mend his universe already.

It wasn't going to happen again.

It was good that he was still feeling flashes of attraction to Isla.

Because, with each one, he was taking a bigger step back.

A week later, the results of all Isla's tests came through. She showed Jake the summary that had been sent by the organ transplant specialists in Auckland.

Jake was blinking at the paper, almost as if he was fighting tears.

'You're pretty much a perfect match,' he said. He sounded surprised. Proud of her, even.

Isla's smile wobbled a little. She'd felt quite emotional when she'd read that, too. For a moment, it had been a wonderful feeling. As if the universe was giving her permission to embrace Arlo as her closest living relative.

Her *family*.

But panic had appeared from its usual hiding place deep inside her and destroyed that warm glow with its sharp claws. Her head promptly quashed what her heart was doing, by reminding her what it was like to have—and then lose—a family that you adored.

Distance…

Keep it clinical. Further towards the impersonal side of this spectrum of involvement. She could still do what was right and be there to support her sister's child in any way she could, as long as she stayed within the boundaries she needed for her personal safety.

'Let's hope it's never needed,' she said. 'But it's an insurance policy, isn't it? How is Arlo today? Is he back at school? Is that why you've come into work?'

Jake shook his head. 'I've got a sitter for him. Lovely young woman who lives on our street and does shift work so she has a day off today.'

'But he's doing okay, isn't he? I thought he was looking well when I came around the other night.'

'He's fine.' Jake nodded. 'A bit quiet, I guess, but that's no surprise. Being sick and in hospital again must have been a nasty reminder of everything he's been through recently. I just don't want to push it. Or for him to go back to school while he's still on the antibiotics. Maybe he'll pick up when the course is finished.'

'A bit of sea air might help. And a change of scene. Maybe you'd both like to come to the beach for a couple of days?'

Isla knew instantly that she'd said the wrong thing. She could actually feel Jake pulling away. Any shared relief at knowing that she was a match if Arlo did need a kidney transplant in the future was evaporating rapidly. Jake did not want to be in her house with its reminders of not only how the attraction between them had exploded into physical contact but how it had almost destroyed what had brought them together in the first place—the future of the young boy that was connected so closely to both of them. The boy whose future they both needed to take responsibility for.

She got that as well.

It hadn't been as hard as she had feared, going into the old villa with that fish and chip dinner for Jake and Arlo a couple of evenings ago. She'd managed to walk past Jake's bedroom and control that shiver of need that was trying to reach every cell in her body. That had been an encouraging step in the right direction. Distance was working its magic. It probably wasn't going to take long at all, thanks to the skills she'd honed years ago. She *would* be able to return to the normal, *safe* life she had built for herself.

Jake handed her back the letter from the transplant team.

'Thanks,' he said. 'I'd love a mini-break at the beach but it's the last thing I should be doing at the moment. I've used up all my sick leave and annual leave and if I don't start making up some shifts I'll be on leave without pay and that's not ideal when I've taken on a mortgage and have a family to support.'

Isla felt herself stiffen. She even took a step back. Was this a reprimand for her lack of substantial enough support?

But Jake was smiling. 'I'm not complaining,' he said. 'I never thought I'd have my own family but here I am with a human kid and a fur child. But if you could have Arlo and Ben to stay for a day and maybe overnight once in a while, it would be a huge help. I could work some double shifts and make up for all the cover Sam's been providing.'

So he wanted her to spend time with Arlo but not himself? That would certainly make it easier to keep the distance between them they were both carefully nurturing, but Isla could almost imagine that the ache in her chest was coming from a small piece of her heart breaking off. Maybe the part that had sprung a crack that time she'd felt left out of the visible bond forming between Jake and Arlo. When she'd had a glimpse of how much better life could be if you weren't lonely.

But if you weren't lonely you had something to lose. Something so precious, just the thought of losing it was enough to make you back away. This was a timely reminder of the reason she needed to do this properly. It might be her last chance to repair her safety barriers before they developed any more cracks and the less time they had in each other's company the better, until this became one hell of a lot easier.

She'd more than contributed to the damage done to the new life being built for Arlo when he'd been so shocked by seeing her kissing his uncle. Some time alone with Arlo and Ben might allow her to help repair his confidence that he was safe from any new major changes in his life. She could back Jake up and confirm that they were friends. That Arlo was the most important person in both their lives and that wasn't about to change.

She managed a much less wobbly smile this time. 'Of course. I've got two days off from Wednesday. If he doesn't mind spending that much time with me, I can collect him as early as you like in the morning and bring him back on Friday when I'm on shift again. And I'd be happy to stay in the house with him over the weekend if you're working then.'

'Really?' It was more than relief in Jake's eyes.

It looked like a mix of both gratitude and hope, and that gave Isla another pang of guilt. How hard had it been for this man who was passionate about his work to have to suddenly juggle parenthood he hadn't chosen to take on? This might have been an emotional minefield for Isla to have been navigating but it was more than that for Jake. Like Samantha, maybe working in a small regional hospital had not been the plan for the rest of his life. Had he sacrificed career ambitions in order to buy a house and settle down for the sake of giving Arlo a solid base? Had he also turned his back on a personal lifestyle where hard work was balanced by the fun of casual, no-strings relationships with women?

He wasn't complaining about it. He never had. He'd taken the responsibility on board and he was giving it his best shot. Isla was seeing the real Jake here. An intelligent, hardworking, passionate, *kind* man who was capable of total commitment. Okay, there'd been that minor hiccup of getting too close to her but that had been done with the absolute intention that it was only going to be a one-off and nobody was going to be hurt by it. Someone had been—Arlo—and she had to own her share of the responsibility for that.

Jake deserved someone in his life who was prepared to be doing a whole lot more.

'We're going to be co-parents,' Isla reminded him. 'It's about time I started doing my fair share.'

It felt good.

Looking in the rearview mirror to catch the dark eyes of the black and white dog who was sitting up so straight. Ben had been waiting for that glance, hadn't he? The hopeful look Isla caught made her smile.

'Okay… You can have the window open.'

She pushed the button on her armrest and, moments later, Ben had his nose in the rush of air outside the car and his ears were back. He looked like he was grinning. A sideways glance was a different story, however. In the front passenger seat, Arlo had his face turned away from Isla. He was either asleep or pretending to be and he stayed that way until she got home.

'What would you like to do first?' Isla asked. 'Shall we take Ben for a walk on the beach? I need to gather a bit of driftwood kindling for the fire and I bet he'd enjoy chasing a few sticks.'

But Arlo shook his head. 'I'm tired,' he said. 'Can I just read my book?'

'Sure.'

Ben looked longingly at the track that led to the beach but plodded faithfully beside Arlo as they went inside. Isla had the horrible feeling that her nephew might choose to go into his bedroom and shut the door to put a physical barrier between them but he chose the window seat in the living area and had his nose buried in his book almost instantly.

'You're up to *The Voyage of the Dawn Treader*? I think that was my absolute favourite. Are you enjoying it?'

Arlo shrugged. 'It's okay.'

If Isla had been hoping for a chance to talk about King Caspian and his search for the seven lost lords of Narnia, she let it go with what felt like relief. Did she really want to be reminded that this story had featured a gorgeous boat out on the wildest seas and she'd read it at least five times? Because she was one of the McGregor girls and she'd been born with seawater for blood?

Given his love of surfing, Isla suspected that Arlo had inherited some of that passion from his mother but, if so, it was well hidden today, along with any sense of connection with her.

Clearly, she had a fair way to go to earn back that embryonic trust that had begun to grow the day they'd built the teepee on the beach and created the private joke about sandy sandwiches. The best thing she could do for now was to leave him in peace to escape into his book and just be here for him. Maybe she could tempt Arlo down to the beach when Ben needed a run.

Isla made herself a cup of tea and settled down at the table to get on with the copy edits of *Code... Revenge*, which was due back on her editor's desk tomorrow. She wanted to read over the last scene particularly carefully. That was where she'd redeemed her damaged hero, Alex. When Riley was lying there, unable to breathe and so terrified and he'd realised how much he loved her and that he couldn't let her die. He breathed for her until the paralytic drug wore off a few minutes later. And then he walked out of the story, with another syringe full of the drug in his hands. It was a poignant ending that was not only fitting, given the way Alex had used his medical knowledge to take so many other lives, but having to deal with it also added to the growth of her heroine, Riley, whose strength shone in the last lines. Her editor had loved it.

She'd finished her work by lunchtime but Arlo didn't want to go outside and he barely touched the BLT sandwiches Isla made for him. When she noticed Ben sitting beside the door, having abandoned the position beside the window seat that he'd been in for hours now, she groaned apologetically.

'Sorry, Ben. You need to go outside, don't you?' She opened the door for him and he shot off into the trees, clearly desperate for a pee. Isla looked over her shoulder. 'Want to come for a quick walk with us? Just for a bit of fresh air?'

Arlo shook his head. 'I've got to a good bit in the book,' he muttered. 'Eustace has just been turned into a dragon.'

Oh… Isla wanted to ask if Aslan had reappeared but she didn't want to be dropping any spoilers. She looked out of the door and caught a flash of Ben's white tail amongst the trees. She should take him down to the beach for a few minutes. Then she looked back at Arlo. She couldn't leave him alone in the house, could she?

With another silent apology to Ben, she called for him to come back into the house.

She waited a moment and then stepped out onto the veranda to call again because she couldn't see him.

'Ben? Here, boy! Time to come back inside.'

She waited another moment and then she put her fingers in her mouth to produce the kind of whistle that Pat Murphy would have used to summon his sheepdog, but there was no response to that call either.

'Arlo, I'm just going down the track a bit to call Ben.

I think he's headed off to the beach by himself. I'll be back in two minutes, okay?'

Arlo nodded but didn't look up from his book.

Isla ran down to the beach. She shaded her eyes from the sun and looked in both directions but could see no sign of Ben. She shouted his name but the only response was for a lone fisherman on the rocks to turn his head.

'Have you seen a black and white dog?'

He shook his head.

'If you do, can you come and tell me? I live just up the track there.'

He nodded this time.

Isla turned and ran back up the track. She shouted for Ben again as she neared the house but she could feel her heart sinking. He must have gone in the other direction. Down the driveway and towards the road. Had he finally done what she'd been afraid he might do and gone looking for the person he must have been missing ever since the night of the accident?

When she got to the corner of the house, she found Arlo standing outside.

'Where is he?' he demanded. 'Where's Ben?'

'He can't be far away.' Isla tried to sound reassuring. 'He wasn't on the beach so I'm going to go looking for him up the driveway and on the road.'

She had no idea what direction the dog might have taken, though. What if he was following his instincts and taking the straightest line possible through hundreds of acres of forest to get to the last place he'd seen Pat? The main highway, with all the dangers that came with fast-moving traffic.

She understood why Arlo was looking so stricken. Ben had been the best thing that could have happened to him when he'd been struggling with the disintegration of his life. Their bond had been palpable from the first moment when she'd seen him sitting there on the edge of that ditch with his arm around the dog.

What was really shocking was that Arlo had tears trickling down his cheeks. She'd never seen him cry. He'd been so shut-off. Self-protective. Keeping his grief so private. A lot like the person she'd become in order to protect herself, and her heart ached for Arlo because she knew what it would have taken to shatter that shell.

'You never wanted me.' His voice was strangled by the depth of emotion it carried. 'I heard you say it—that you didn't want me to live with you. Uncle Jake never wanted me either. Not really. He likes *you* more than me. I saw him kissing you. I'm just in the way. Ben's the only one who loves me and…' the sob that escaped was completely heartbroken '…and now *he's* gone…'

CHAPTER TWELVE

JAKE'S PHONE WAS on silent but he felt the vibration of an incoming call and a quick glance told him it was from Isla. He couldn't answer it, however, because he had just entered the cubicle occupied by a woman who'd come in with a four-day history of abdominal pain, fever and vomiting.

He had to suppress the flash of worry that Isla might be ringing because of some concern over Arlo.

'Have you had any episodes like this before, Beth?'

'Yes. Once.' The middle-aged woman was pale and there were beads of perspiration on her forehead. She was lying back on the bed, her knees slightly bent, with a vomit container firmly clutched in one hand as Jake adjusted the blanket and her hospital gown to expose her stomach for an abdominal examination.

'How long ago?'

'It was last year.'

'Did you go and see your GP?' Jake could see that Beth's stomach was slightly bloated.

'No.' Beth groaned. 'We'd been to Auckland for the weekend and we went and had a fast food feast. *Big* mistake and not just because it broke my diet. I thought

I deserved to suffer and learn my lesson and it went away after a couple of days.'

Jake nodded. Beth's gender, age and weight issues were adding to first impressions that this was a case of cholecystitis caused by gallstones. He unhooked his stethoscope from around his neck. 'I'm just going to listen to your stomach for a minute.'

As expected, he couldn't hear normal bowel sounds.

'Can you point to where the pain is worst?'

Beth touched the right upper quadrant of her abdomen so Jake started his palpation in the lower left. Again, he had to shove away the thought that maybe Arlo was also experiencing abdominal pain and that might be due to a deterioration of his kidney's condition. Becoming a parent was changing every aspect of his life, wasn't it? Including his work. But it was easier to put the concerning thought aside this time.

Arlo was with Isla and Jake trusted her completely. He was sure she cared about Arlo as much as he did, even if she was still too afraid to acknowledge that. She would know exactly what to do if Arlo wasn't well and if she was at all worried she'd bring him back here to the emergency department so that he could be checked.

He left palpating the most painful area of Beth's abdomen until last but she stiffened and groaned almost before he'd touched it.

'That paracetamol hasn't helped the pain much, has it?'

'No.'

'I'm going to get an IV line in now. We need to take some blood tests and then we'll get some fluids up because you're dehydrated from not eating and drinking and all this vomiting. I'm going to give you something stronger for the pain and we'll see if we can get that nausea under control for you as well.'

As soon as Beth was more comfortable and while he waited for blood results and for the portable ultrasound machine to become available, Jake went into the unoccupied staffroom to return Isla's call.

'*Jake*...'

Just the way she said his name revealed how upset Isla was and Jake felt a beat of fear.

'What is it?' he asked. 'What's happened? Is it Arlo?'

'No. Yes... I mean no, he's fine physically but...' He could hear that Isla was moving. A door clicked shut. Did she not want Arlo to be hearing this? He heard the gulp of Isla's inward breath. 'Ben's gone missing.'

'What?'

'I let him out to pee and...he disappeared. I went down to the beach but he wasn't there and a fisherman said he hadn't seen him. I came back to the house and found Arlo was beside himself. We've been searching for the last hour or more—up the driveway and along to Sailors Grave beach. We met some surfers there but they said they hadn't seen any dogs at all.'

'Where do you think he could have gone?'

'I'm worried that he might have tried to go back to his old home and find Pat. Our local ambo told me he lived not far north from here. I think I need to get in the car and go looking but...oh, *God*, Jake. I can't leave Arlo here alone, but what if I take him with me and Ben's on the road somewhere and he's been...'

He knew what she couldn't bring herself to say. That they might find Ben had been hit by a car and killed. That the emotional storm of trying to be with Arlo and navigate yet another loss would be more than she could handle.

'He's a smart dog,' he said. 'I'm sure he knows how to keep himself safe around roads.'

Isla didn't seem reassured. 'There's something worse,' she told him. 'He did hear us. That first morning when we were talking about who was going to look after Ben.'

Jake blinked very slowly. That was when he'd said that he couldn't have a dog in his apartment, wasn't it? When he was so dismayed by Isla's reluctance to be involved with her nephew. He could remember snatches of that tense conversation.

'*You think it's going to be easy for me to take on the unexpected responsibility of raising a child? And maybe caring for a dog?*'

'*He can't* live *here.*' How appalled had Isla been? '*Any more than Ben can. It's. Not. Possible.*'

Isla was sounding equally appalled right now. 'He said…he said that neither of us really wanted him and—you were right—seeing us kissing had made him feel like he was in the way and that you liked me more than him. He even said…' Isla had to clear her throat to continue '…that Ben's the only one who loves him.'

Jake swallowed. Hard. 'He doesn't really believe that,' he said. 'He's just upset. Look… I've got a patient with probable cholecystitis. I've paged Doug who's on call for surgery and as soon as I've done an ultrasound

I'll be able to hand her over and I can get away to come and help. Take Arlo and drive up to where Pat used to live and…call me back after that. I might not be able to answer straight away but I'll get back to you just as soon as I can, I promise.'

'Okay…' Isla's voice sounded small.

Frightened. Jake knew perfectly well how strong this woman was and that she could cope with whatever needed to be done but, dear Lord…he was gripped by an almost overwhelming longing to be closer to her. Close enough to take her into his arms and hold her tightly enough to be able to infuse her with some of his own strength.

To hold her against his heart for long enough to let her know how important she was to him. How much he cared about *her* as well as Arlo.

'Isla?'

'Yes?'

'We can deal with this. Whatever happens, we'll get through this. All of us. Together.'

It wasn't what he really wanted to say. That was still trapped in his head. Or his heart?

We'll get through this, Isla. I love you. It's going to be okay…

But maybe Isla hadn't heard anything anyway. There was only silence when he finished speaking and Jake didn't know when she had ended the call.

Beth Fielding's blood results were back and, along with her rising temperature, they were adding up to confirming Jake's provisional diagnosis of gallbladder inflammation caused by a blockage from gallstones. All that was needed now was an ultrasound.

'This'll be a bit cold,' he warned as he squeezed gel onto Beth's bare skin.

He pressed the transducer into position and angled it, waiting for the shapes on the screen to settle into something recognisable so he could get his bearings, but it was taking longer than it should. He had to focus. If he let his patient down because he was worried about something he couldn't actually do anything about right now, he would be failing everyone. Beth, his colleagues and…the people he cared most about in the world.

Isla and Arlo.

And…yeah… Ben, too.

They were a family, weren't they?

All of them.

Jake gave himself a mental shake and concentrated fully on what was coming into view as he shifted the angle of the transducer he was holding. The gallbladder was enlarged and there was fluid accumulating around it. The surgeon, Doug, came into the cubicle as he was starting to catch the outline of a stone that looked like it was firmly blocking the bile duct.

'Bingo,' Doug said, peering at the screen. He nodded. 'I think we might be taking your gallbladder out as soon as possible, Beth. We don't want this happening again, do we?'

With his patient admitted and transferred to the ward, Jake was watching and waiting for a call from Isla. It was over an hour after she'd first called him that his phone buzzed again.

'Hey...' He didn't waste time on greetings. 'Any luck?'

'No.' She sounded utterly defeated. 'Arlo went into his bedroom as soon as we got back and he slammed the door shut. I was trying to think of what to do next when someone turned up at the front door.'

Oh, *no*... Jake's heart was sinking like a stone.

'It was that fisherman I'd seen when I first went down to check the beach. He told me he'd been packing up his gear and he thought he'd seen Ben. Out on the rocks.'

'He *thought* he'd seen him?'

'He saw something. He'd turned his head and caught a glimpse of something black and white, but a big wave had come in and washed over the rocks and whatever it was had vanished. He couldn't be a hundred percent sure, but he thought he should warn me.' Isla's sigh was heartfelt. 'I walked up the driveway with him because I needed time to think but I'm nearly back at the house now. How on earth am I going to tell Arlo? This is going to be devastating for him.'

'Wait until I get there. We can do it together.'

Her voice was only a whisper now. 'I thought I could keep myself safe by not getting too close but...it hasn't worked. I care too much, Jake and... I don't know what to do.'

'You do,' Jake said softly. 'You just need to listen to what's in your heart.'

But Isla didn't seem to be listening to him.

'And then there's *you*,' she added.

'*Me?*' For a wild moment Jake thought that Isla was going to confess that she cared too much about *him*.

The way he was feeling about *her*?

But Isla wasn't saying anything. Had she hung up on him again?

'Are you still there?'

'Um…yeah… I'm here. I'm on the veranda.'

'What's wrong?'

'Did you put Arlo's surfboard anywhere else? Like in the shed with the kayaks?'

'No. Why?'

'It's not here. His wetsuit's gone off the hook too and…oh, *no*…his bedroom window's open.'

Jake's blood was running cold. Had Arlo been eavesdropping again? Did he already know that Ben might have drowned?

'Can you see through the window? Is he in his room?'

'No.'

'*Go*,' Jake urged. '*Run*. Get down to the beach. Don't hang up…'

He could hear the crunch of her feet on the shells and twigs that lined the track down to the beach. He could hear her breathing, harsh and rapid as she ran as fast as she could. And then he could hear her voice over the wash of breaking waves.

'Arlo? *Arlo?*'

The wait was unbearable.

'Can you see anything?'

'The surf's too big. The tide's right in. And the light's fading. It's…'

Another silence with only the sound of the waves and Isla still trying to catch her breath.

'*There*… I think…*yes*, there it is again—a flash of

red. That has to be his surfboard. Oh, my God, Jake…
Arlo's in the sea. Out near that sea stack island…'

Fear had morphed into the kind of calm determination that came with taking control of a life and death situation. Jake knew exactly what he needed to do.

'Stay right where you are, Isla,' he instructed. 'I'm getting help on the way.'

He had to end the call so that he could call the emergency services.

'Police,' he said to the person who answered the call and asked which service he required. 'And Search and Rescue. This is *urgent*…'

What was worse?

The fear of losing yet another person she loved to drowning?

Or facing her worst fear and getting into a raging sea herself?

But Isla was almost distracted from her personal fear of the ocean by the realisation that she was admitting how much she cared about Arlo.

She *did* love him.

Of course she did. He'd captured her heart from the instant she'd seen that cheeky smile and recognised her sister in his face. She'd felt the bond of family when that first numbness of grief began wearing off, despite doing her best to deny it.

He was just a kid but he'd been brave enough to go into this surf to try and save a dog that *he* loved. A dog who'd been by his side in some of the worst moments of his life. Who'd loved him back with every fibre of his being, the way that only dogs could do.

In the end, Isla didn't even acknowledge her fear. She peeled off her jeans and kicked off her shoes to get rid of the weight they'd add when they were wet. She waded into the ocean, wishing she had a board to help get her past the breaking waves. She had to dive through them to stop herself being knocked over and pushed back to shore, or worse, pinned underwater.

And then she was swimming. For the first time in five years, she was swimming but it felt like only yesterday that she'd been desperately battling the swells of icy seawater. She found herself thinking of teaching Sage to cope with swimming in the open sea.

Stay calm. Panic will steal your energy.

Short, choppy strokes to get through the swells, longer ones in the lulls.

Control your breathing, quick sideways turns of your head. Float on your back if you need a few deep breaths or to gather strength...

And then the mantra—*a big wave is a challenge, not a wall.*

The light was almost gone but, at the top of the swells, Isla could see the island clearly enough to not lose focus on her goal. It wasn't that far but it felt as if it took forever. And then she could see the flash of colour amongst the rocks at the base of the sea stack's cliff. Red and green. Watermelon colours. She put on a burst of speed, but that was a mistake because she was too close now and the rocks weren't far below the surface. The knock and scrape on her ankle made her cry out in pain.

'*Isla?*'

She could hear the fear in Arlo's voice. Or was it fear?

'Stay there!' Arlo yelled. 'I'll bring you my board.'

And, moments later, there he was. This astonishingly courageous nine-year-old boy who paddled towards her on his ridiculously pretty surfboard and then they both used it as a float to get over the sharp rocks and out of the water. It was Arlo who led the way between rocks to get to a small ledge on the cliff of the sea stack, where he put the board down.

It was only then that Isla, shivering uncontrollably now, could give in to the relief of finding Arlo alive. Were they tears streaming down her face or was it the seawater from her hair? Not that it mattered. Or maybe it did. Because if she could cry again, she was feeling things. *Everything.*

'I'm s-so happy to s-see you,' she said to Arlo. 'I love you s-so much.'

She would never be able to remember whether she held her arms out first or to catch Arlo as he threw himself into them. That didn't matter either. They clung to each other and they were both crying.

'Ben's here,' Arlo told her. 'He's okay…'

He was. He squeezed onto the ledge with them and in the huddle of three bodies Isla could feel the tiniest bit of warmth beginning to penetrate her frozen skin.

'What do we do now, Isla?'

'We wait,' she said. 'We stay right here where we're safe and we wait for help to come.'

'Will it come soon?'

'Yes.' Isla could say that with the utmost confidence. 'Your Uncle Jake's on his way. He knows where we are.'

And he was her hero. Because he was doing whatever he could right now to get help to them. Because he'd taken Arlo into his life without hesitation and was prepared to change his entire life to care for a lost boy who was his family. Because he'd found her and brought Arlo into *her* life. It would never be the same again. It would be so much better.

Okay…maybe she had been keeping herself safe by creating that distance between herself and anybody else, but she'd been cutting herself off from real life, hadn't she? The only emotion she'd allowed herself was channelled through the characters in her books. She'd allowed her loss and her grief to turn into walls. Maybe that mantra was true about more than scarily big waves in the sea and other things in life should be seen as challenges and not walls. Good grief…she'd even convinced herself that her attraction to Jake was due to a physical need when the truth was so much bigger.

When her love for Jake—as well as Arlo—was so much bigger than she'd allowed herself to see.

She needed him now.

They all did.

The rescue helicopter had touched down in the field beside Coromandel Hospital just long enough to allow Jake to jump on board. They might need a doctor, he'd told the emergency services. And he knew exactly where they needed to search. Sam had found some search and rescue gear for him and he covered his own clothes with the bright orange overalls.

'Wish I could go with you,' she said. 'I'm winch trained. That might be useful.'

'There won't be enough room,' he said. 'Sorry, there's no way I'm not going. This is my family.'

'I know.' Sam gave him a hug as they heard the helicopter coming in to land. 'Good luck. I really hope everyone's okay.'

'You and me both,' Jake said grimly.

The helicopter crew gave him a helmet and showed him how to do up his safety straps. Moments later they were flying over the dark, forest-covered hills towards the east coast of the peninsula.

'It's Otara Bay,' he told them. 'Next bay around from Sailors Grave. There's a tall island just out from the shore. Rocks around the bottom, steep cliffs and some trees on the top. That's where the surfboard was spotted.'

Isla's phone had rung only once and gone to voicemail when he'd tried it as soon as he'd hung up from alerting the emergency services. Had she been trying to call him? Or was the phone broken? Deep down, Jake thought he knew what might have happened, despite him telling Isla to stay where she was on the beach.

He would have done the same thing himself.

Gone into the sea.

To try and save Arlo.

And it wouldn't have been because he was trying to make up for not having saved his brother. It would have been because he loved Arlo *that* much.

It was completely dark by the time they started tracking up the coast to Otara Bay. When they got close to the coordinates of their destination, they activated the night sun on the bottom of the helicopter that lit up the ground beneath them like the brightest spotlight ever.

'That's the car park and toilets for Sailors Grave.' Jake pointed as he looked out of the window on his side. 'And that's Isla's house. It's straight from there to the beach and then straight out to the island.'

The helicopter hovered over the beach. There was no one to be seen. Then the pilot did a tight turn and Jake got a close-up view of how wild the surf was—the foam a stark white against the oily black of the seawater in the glare of the night sun.

The voice of a crew member cut through the spike of his rising fear.

'There… Four o'clock. On the side of the cliff, just above the rocks.'

'Roger that.' The pilot did another turn and then began hovering directly over the island.

Jake leaned to peer out of the window on the other side and in the intense light he could see two very pale faces well below them. And…yes…between the huddle of the woman and the boy, there was the black and white shape of Ben the border collie.

Plans were being made. They were going to touch down on the beach and Jake would jump out and then a crewman would be winched down to where Isla and Arlo were sheltering. Because it was such a short distance to shore, they would be put in a nappy harness, strapped to the crewman and taken to shore. Jake could check them and if any medical attention was needed, they would land on the beach and take them on board to go back to Thames.

'Can you rescue the dog, too?' he asked before he jumped out and followed the instructions to keep his head well down as he ran clear of the rotors. 'Please? It's *really* important.'

He didn't hear any response. All he could do was stand on the beach in the dark, with only the crashing waves for company, and watch as the helicopter was positioned again out to sea and the crew got on with what they were so good at doing.

Finally, he saw the figure leaning out from the open door on the side of the aircraft and then dropping slowly towards the sea and then sideways towards the island. It seemed to take a very long time to get things sorted for the first rescue, but then the larger shape of two people locked together rose a short distance above the sea and came towards where Jake was standing.

The larger of the two figures got their feet on the beach and unhooked his harness. It was only then that Jake realised Arlo had been the first to be rescued and he held his arms out to gather his nephew as close to him as he could. He'd wrap one of the foil blankets he'd been left with around Arlo in just a minute. This hug was too important to postpone.

He was still holding Arlo, now enveloped in foil, as the helicopter came towards them again. Jake was expecting it to be Isla this time so it was a shock when he saw that it wasn't. It was Ben.

'She wouldn't let me take her first,' the crewman shouted. 'Said she wasn't going to risk losing him again. Not when he was a member of the family.'

Ben was soaked. Jake wrapped the dog in a foil blanket as well and Arlo knelt on the sand beside him to keep it from blowing away in the downdraught from the helicopter.

And then they waited again. Jake felt as if his heart was in his mouth this time. He watched the figure touch down on the island and he could see the movements as Isla stepped into the harness and was clipped to the crewman and the winch line. He watched as she was lifted into the air and swept towards him and when her feet finally hit the sand he had forgotten he should have a foil blanket ready for her to be wrapped in. All he wanted to wrap her in was himself. He needed to gather Isla into his arms. Into his life and into his future. He wasn't going to metaphorically swallow his heart again, he was going to take it and offer it to Isla.

And Arlo. And Ben. If ever there was a package deal, this was it.

Maybe he should have been worried about Isla not being ready to accept what was on offer. Or not wanting her life to change that much. But he wasn't worried at all. Because, as Isla ran towards them, he could see that she wanted this as much as he did.

And then he felt a small arm around his waist. Arlo, with Ben by his side, had his other arm out, ready to catch Isla. So Jake put one arm over Arlo's shoulders and held the other one out and they were making a semicircle that they closed into a full circle as soon as Isla got close enough.

The tightest circle ever.

It was a wonder Ben didn't get squashed in the middle of it.

EPILOGUE

Five years later

THE LEAN BLACK-CLAD FIGURE on the surfboard was skimming the lip of a big wave at Sailors Grave beach.

He launched himself and his board into the air and then twisted a full three-hundred-and-sixty degree circle before landing back on the wave. It was a trick that required the technical skills of precise timing, speed control and balance and Arlo had been practising it for weeks, in the hope of using it to impress the judges at the surf event he would be competing in this summer. This was the first time he hadn't wiped out in an attempt to conquer it.

Thank goodness Jake and Isla hadn't missed it, which was a small miracle given that they were trying to watch their two-year-old twins, Tayla and Harley, who were sitting where only the very ends of the waves could foam around their chubby legs. They shrieked with glee as the foam came close enough to be smacked with the palms of their hands or the little plastic spades they were trying to use between waves to fill buckets with sand and make a castle.

Ben, too elderly a dog now to want to be in the middle of the action, was sitting far enough away to avoid being splashed or hit with spades. Not too far, though. He had been watching over and protecting these babies from the moment their proud parents had brought them home from the hospital.

They both turned to each other to share a delighted grin after seeing the fist-pump Arlo pushed into the air as he rode the rest of that wave with the joy of knowing he'd succeeded.

They shared a long, loving glance as well. One of probably a million such glances they'd shared ever since the night of that dramatic rescue of both Arlo and Ben. The night they'd told each other how much in love with each other they were. The night they'd promised to share the rest of their lives. The night they'd made a vow to respect the past but make the most of all the joy the future could bring them.

Arlo came in to shore when his wave faded into foam and ran towards them through the shallows with his board under one arm.

'Did you *see* that?'

'We sure did, mate.' Jake gave Arlo a fist-bump. 'It was *awesome*.'

'I'm so proud of you.' Isla's smile felt as if it reached from one ear to the other. 'What did it feel like?'

Arlo shook seawater from his spiky dark hair and bent over to focus on unwrapping his ankle cuff to detach the leg rope. He was a teenage boy, and Isla should have known how embarrassing it was to talk about feelings. Having dropped his board on the sand, however, he turned his head far enough to give her a grin.

That cheeky grin that she loved so much. The one that made her remember Sage. With love. As much love as she had for her sister's son.

'Like flying,' Arlo said. 'It was *so* cool.'

Harley was getting to his feet with all the determination of a very mobile toddler. He bypassed his parents and went straight to Arlo.

'Swim,' he demanded, holding up his arms.

Tayla wasn't far behind him. 'Me,' she pleaded. 'Me, too.'

Arlo picked up Harley and walked out to where the water was about knee-deep between waves. He held Harley under his armpits and dipped him so he could kick his legs underwater and then lifted him swiftly as the next wave rolled in at greater than head height. Isla was pretty sure her babies had inherited a genetic love for the ocean because this was a game that both twins had adored since their very first visit to the beach.

It was Jake who picked up Tayla so that she could share the fun. Isla was happy to stay on the sand, letting the waves caress her ankles, feeling the sun on her skin and smelling the salt in the air. Moments like these were the best.

Sheer joy. Her heart was so filled with it that it almost brought tears to her eyes.

They hadn't brought a picnic lunch to the beach. Why would they, when they could walk along the track and back to their house and have sandwiches that didn't have any sand in them?

They lived in the old villa in Thames now. Isla was still on maternity leave but she was seriously considering not going back to join Jake in the emergency department of Coromandel Hospital. She was loving being a parent to babies again. And her fans were crying out for another Tessa Townsend medical thriller. There wasn't time to do everything and she had to make some choices. As much as she loved working with her husband, she loved being a mother and an aunt and a writer and a homemaker even more.

Okay…maybe she could just do a day here and there. So that she could enjoy watching Jake's brilliance. And get a few ideas for her next story?

Ben gave up standing between Isla and the splashing toddlers. He came back to stand beside her. She looked down and smiled as she met the dog's dark eyes. She always knew exactly what he was thinking and he was totally on board with her having more time to spend with him.

With her family.

With the man she loved so much that she couldn't imagine her life without Jake in it. With Arlo, who had been the one who'd pushed her past those barriers she'd built that had kept this kind of joy out of her life. He had made this possible.

To be married again.

To be a *mother* again.

To be a family. For ever.

* * * * *

*Look out for the next story in
the Coastside ER miniseries*

Single Dad for the Daredevil Doctor

*And if you enjoyed this story, check out these other
great reads from Alison Roberts*

Single Dad's Christmas Wish
Their Fake Date Rescue
Midwife's Three-Date Rule

All available now!

SINGLE DAD FOR THE DAREDEVIL DOCTOR

ALISON ROBERTS

MILLS & BOON

CHAPTER ONE

YES…!

Everyone in Coromandel Hospital's emergency department knew Samantha Gillespie was an adrenaline junkie and that was probably why they were shaking their heads but had a tolerant smile on their faces as she rushed past them to get to the staff locker rooms.

Another doctor, her friend Isla, looked up from where she was stitching a cut on a patient's finger. 'You're in a hurry, Sam. It's not a LandSAR callout, is it?'

'Yes.' Sam wasn't slowing down. 'Bunch of five- to seven-year-olds on a school trip to see Kauri trees in the Forest Park up towards the Pinnacles. There's been a flash flood that's turned a creek into a roaring torrent. Some of the youngest ones have been cut off and the weather's turning. Jake's covering for me.' She was far enough away now to have to raise her voice to be heard.

'Good luck!' Isla called back. 'We'll be on standby for any incoming.'

Sam threw open her locker seconds later and reached for the neat pile of clothing at the bottom—her official Land Search and Rescue team member gear. She swapped her scrub pants for the waterproof tactical-style pants with all the pockets and straps for things like her headlamp and snack bars, a water bottle and GPS device. A long-sleeved merino top replaced her tunic and her sneakers were discarded in favour of hiking boots. She shrugged on a bright orange jacket and picked up a matching beanie that would keep her wayward dark waves under more control than a scrunchie could achieve in a fierce wind, pulling it onto her head to leave her hands free to reach for something more important—the backpack with all the medical gear she might need to stabilise someone who could be critically injured or sick.

The next stop was the securely locked cabinet in the supply room to add what couldn't be kept in her locker. She gathered supplies swiftly, adding the restricted drugs like potent painkillers and sedatives. She ran an eye over the kits in her pack that she'd restocked after her last callout. Dressings and splints, IV supplies and airway equipment. She grabbed a few more packets that contained foil blankets. Were these trapped kids adequately dressed for being outside in New Zealand's rugged landscape for a much longer time than had been expected for their school outing?

Was anybody injured? Or worse, washed away by the creek and now missing and unlikely to have survived?

She'd find out soon enough because she was good to go.

Taking a deep breath, Sam slipped her arms through the straps of the backpack and walked out of the supply room, now completely focused on what might be waiting for her.

In the zone.

Happy.

Well…happy wasn't anywhere near the right word for how she was feeling but she *was* in, if not her happiest place, a part of her life that the most significant because it brought together the two things she lived for—medicine and a possibly challenging physical adventure. This was the place where she felt energised and so…alive. This was her purpose in life and anticipation—excitement, even—was flooding her veins like a drug. She walked swiftly through the reception area towards the front doors of this regional hospital, aware that heads were turning and expressions were impressed that one of the doctors here was involved with such a well-respected rescue organisation. That she could, in fact, be putting herself in danger to help other people whose lives might be at risk.

The thought that she could be putting herself in danger wasn't an issue for Sam. If anything, it added to this delicious anticipation. How shocked would any of these people who were watching her be if they knew just how much danger Sam Gillespie had thrived on in her teenage years? How reckless she'd been? Nobody blinked an eye, however, at the idea that a doctor who chose to work on the frontline of healthcare in an emergency department might also want to be involved in the thrill of *really* being out on the frontline. In the wild. Riding shotgun with specialist rescue teams into flood-stricken areas or earthquake zones, perhaps, or heading out to sea with the coastguard or deep underground in a cave system.

Sam was ready for anything. She'd tried living without the thrill of a regular adrenaline rush and it wasn't for her. She was ready to embrace any opportunity to jump into a helicopter or ride out with paramedics in an ambulance, beacons flashing and sirens on as they raced to a scene with unknown elements of risk possibly around the very next corner. Or just into a mud-spattered, sturdy four-by-four like the one she knew was waiting for her outside the doors of Coromandel Hospital, ready to whisk her off and into the operation already underway under the organisational umbrella of the local police force.

Sam's expression might have been completely serious as she stepped outside the safety of the hospital and its well-equipped and staffed emergency department but there was a smile lurking deep inside her that she could feel all the way to her bones.

Bring it on…

It was a perfectly ordinary Wednesday afternoon in the Karaka Medical Centre just up the road from Coromandel Hospital.

Dr Adam Carter was signing a prescription for one of his elderly patients who needed a three-month repeat on the blister pack of medications for her high blood pressure, high cholesterol, angina and Type Two diabetes.

'Take this into the pharmacy, Mrs Morrison. They should have a new pack ready for you well before you run out.'

'Yes…it was them who rang me to say it was time to come and see you again and make sure nothing needed to be changed. I feel very well looked after.'

'We do our best,' Adam said. Janet Morrison was well into her nineties but still lived independently in her own home. He'd been her doctor ever since he'd started his career here as a general practitioner, more than ten years ago now, but he'd known her for as long as he could remember because she'd been his grandmother's next-door neighbour.

The soft buzz of a silenced phone against the wooden

top of his desk made Adam glance down. It was his daughter's school calling.

'Excuse me,' he said, smiling to soften an abrupt dismissal of his patient. 'But I'll have to take this call.'

He could feel the beat of concern as he reached for the device. Was the junior school back from the much-anticipated forest outing to see the Kauri trees already? Was there a reason why Charlotte might need picking up before the bell rang for the end of the day's classes?

'Of course.' Mrs Morrison was on her feet with surprising agility and already heading for the door. 'I won't take up another minute of your valuable time.'

Adam swiped the screen of his phone. Thirty seconds later he was following the route Mrs Morrison had taken out of his office, moving so fast he almost bumped into his most senior colleague.

'Derek, could you cover my last two appointments? It's Charlie.' He knew that his face would be communicating the urgency of getting away.

'Of course.' Derek was walking with him towards Reception. 'Is it anything I can help with?'

Adam shook his head. 'There's been a flash flood up near the Pinnacles and it got far enough to disrupt the school's trip to the forest. I don't even know if Charlie's amongst the kids who've been cut off but I have to get up there. The police have been called in. And LandSAR. There's a rescue helicopter on its way from Auckland.'

This was all serious enough that Adam had to pause for a moment as he got outside the medical centre buildings. He put his hand on the roof of his car before he wrenched the driver's door open for just long enough to take a steadying breath and try and quell the kind of fear he'd almost forgotten. The kind he'd had when Charlie had been born so prematurely and he'd spent the hours and days and weeks with that cloud of despair hovering in the background, laden with the fear that he might lose the precious scrap of life that was his daughter.

His medical training hadn't really helped during that fraught time because he'd known too much and could overthink every blip on a monitor or spike in a vital sign measurement. Mind you, he knew almost nothing about search and rescue protocols and just how far or fast a creek could rise in a flash flood and that wasn't helping either. He was still overthinking. Was it like a small tsunami? Big enough that a slightly undersized five-year-old kid couldn't possibly stay upright and might be swept onto rocks or down a waterfall?

He started the car and accelerated as he turned onto the road. Charlie had been so excited about this trip. She'd only started school recently and this was the first adventure with her classmates and the teacher she adored, Miss Kempsey. His offer to go as a parent had been politely declined, thanks to Charlotte Carter's newfound independence in being a schoolgirl. Adam had been hearing all about Kauri trees for weeks now.

He could hear Charlie's voice as he drove to the parking area near the start of the walking track into the Coromandel Forest Park.

'Did you know, Daddy, that Kauri trees can live for hundreds and hundreds of years and grow this big?' Her skinny arms had been outstretched and her fingers spread like starfish. *'We're going to see one. We're going to hold hands with each other and see if it takes the whole class*

to make a circle around the trunk and Miss Kempsey is going to take a photo to go in the school newsletter.'

'I did know how big they are, peanut. They're amazing trees. There's one called Tāne Mahuta, which means "god of the forest". They think it might be two and a half thousand years old and it's over fifty metres tall.'

'Miss Kempsey says they're a ta...ta—' The way Charlie screwed up her nose to think hard was just adorable. 'It's something for Māori people.'

'A taonga? A treasure?'

'Yes.'

Big brown eyes had shone with delight and Adam could feel that surge of love that always turned up when he was around his little girl. The one that had made him pull her close for a squeezy hug.

'You know what?'

'What, Daddy?'

'You're a taonga, too, that's what...'

The parking area was large but there were very few spaces left to put his car. There was a bus, with a long line of children waiting to climb aboard, presumably to be taken back to school. Adam's intent gaze raked the queue and it took only seconds for his heart to sink like a stone as he realised that Charlie was not amongst them. Several police cars were there as well, along with vehicles like utes and Jeeps—the kind that could be used over any kind of terrain for farmwork, or rescue missions.

There was a cluster of people wearing bright orange jackets with a yellow panel on the back and the words SEARCH AND RESCUE in bold black letters. They were checking radios that were being handed out or had their heads bent over maps. Someone tapped a map and then pointed up at a helicopter that was circling some distance away, the sound of its rotors adding another dimension to the tension of the scene.

A policeman came towards Adam as soon as he got out of his car.

'Sorry, sir, but we're asking any parents or other civilians to stay at the school. Most of the children are heading back there now.'

'My daughter isn't with them. She was on this trip and—' He had to clear his throat. 'She's the youngest child in the school. She only turned five a few weeks ago.'

'We're about to start looking for anyone that's not accounted for. We're still asking you to go to the school to wait. I know it's difficult but we'll keep you informed every step of the way.'

'I know this area,' Adam told him. 'I used to go camping in this part of the forest with my mates. And I'm a doctor. I want to help.'

The police officer's expression changed. 'We've already got a doctor from the hospital in the LandSAR team. A Dr Gillespie. Do you know her?'

'I don't think we've met, no.'

'Come and meet her now. But it'll be up to them, and the scene commander, whether it's okay for you to join the search.'

The weather system that had unexpectedly dropped the deluge of water onto where the headwaters of the streams and rivers in the area originated in the mountains was now reaching the lower levels of the Forest Park. Clouds were gathering and mist was swirling around the dramatic jagged peaks of the Pinnacles on the horizon. There were spits of rain and the wind was picking up.

Sam tucked her hair firmly under the hem of her beanie and pulled on a pair of gloves, ready to get moving and start the trek towards where the group of six children had gone missing, along with one of the teachers. But then she stopped dead in her tracks. The scene commander was walking straight towards her, along with the leader of the LandSAR team, Colin Smythe. They weren't alone.

A tall, broad-shouldered man was walking with them and as inappropriate as it was in a situation like this, Sam was momentarily distracted. This stranger looked as though he had walked straight off a movie set or some other kind of world stage because he had to be *the* most astonishingly good-looking man Sam had ever seen in her entire life. She actually glanced behind him, expecting to see a camera crew in his wake. Was he a celebrity, perhaps, who happened to be here scouting a backdrop for a new *Indiana Jones* kind of movie? Or an international journalist who'd got wind of a potentially tragic story about vulnerable children trapped by a rising river?

'This is Dr Adam Carter,' the scene commander told her. 'Local GP.'

Really? Sam had never met him. She'd sure as hell remember if she had. And if he wasn't normally involved with callouts like these, what was he doing here?

'Hi.' Sam's greeting was brief. Cool. 'Good to meet you.'

Was he planning to hang around in the parking area in case more medical assistance was needed? It could be some time before they got anyone back this far and

Sam knew an ambulance was already on its way to be on standby.

'Adam's an experienced tramper,' Colin put in. 'And he knows this area like the back of his hand.'

'Ah…'

If Colin was happy with the doctor's credentials, another medic on the team would be welcome as far as Sam was concerned but his next piece of information made her blink.

'His daughter Charlotte is one of the missing children.' The quirk of his eyebrow acknowledged what he knew she would be thinking. 'You get the final say in whether he joins us or not.'

Sam's gaze flicked back to the stranger and when she met his gaze for more than a heartbeat she saw it. The absolute determination to find his child. The desperate need to be involved. Normally, this would be a red flag that someone might not be able to be part of a team or follow instructions but this man wasn't anything like the distraught family members she'd seen arriving at rescue scenes. Adam Carter had the kind of calmness she recognised—one that had been honed from having to stay in control to deal with life-or-death emergencies. He might be far more personally involved in this situation than any other searcher but Sam's instincts told her that he could still be trusted not to create complications. And that was impressive.

'Come with me,' she said. 'I'll help you grab some gear.' She led the way to a trailer that had LandSAR supplies and quickly located some waterproof over-trousers and a jacket. She also found him a radio.

'Have you used one of these before?'

'Yes.'

'Okay. LandSAR's on channel four. It's six to tune into the police comms but Colin will make sure we're kept informed of any updates. We're hoping the guys on the chopper will spot something soon so we'll know where to head first.'

'Thanks.' The glance at Sam was very direct as he pulled on the trousers. 'How come I haven't met you before? I'm often up at the hospital.'

'I'm fairly new in town,' Sam responded. 'I was a GP up north for a while but I've spent the last few years retraining as an emergency specialist. I'm doing locums while I continue my training and until I've logged enough experience to get my dream job.'

'Which is?' Not that Adam sounded particularly interested in Sam's career ambitions. Of course he wasn't. His daughter was missing. Maybe he was simply being polite. Filling in the time it took to pull the waterproof trousers over his chinos. Or making a vain attempt to distract himself from his fear?

But Sam looked up to where the bright yellow helicopter was still making big circles over what was probably an impenetrably thick canopy of forest trees.

'I want to be on one of those,' she said. 'Preferably as a permanent crew member.'

Adam was zipping up his jacket as both their radios crackled into life.

'Colin to Sam. Are you receiving?'

Sam pushed the button on her radio. 'Loud and clear.'

'All set?'

Sam took out a small backpack that was a basic trauma kit and threw it to Adam.

'On our way. Over and out.'

* * *

The group kept up a steady pace as the track wound up-hill. There were rocks and tree roots to watch out for and Adam imagined how hard this had been for Charlotte. When they'd come for walks in the forest he'd always given her a piggyback over the difficult sections but he could bet she'd insisted on doing this by herself today. He hadn't been on this particular track for many years but he knew there was a short suspension bridge over the creek ahead of them. That would be such an adventure for small children, too. Would Charlie have been scared of the way it swung as she walked across it, clinging to the steel cables that formed the sides of the flexible bridge?

Adam would have been across it in a flash, no matter how hard it was swinging. Except…that it wasn't there now. There were cables still attached to the trees and one that went across the creek but other wires and cables had snapped and the wooden slats of the bridge had been washed away. The bank of the creek had been gouged out on both sides, leaving a slippery stretch of mud and the flow of water across big boulders in the middle was strong enough to be creating waves and some menacing-looking whirlpools.

'At least the water level's dropping,' Colin said. 'But it's still too much of a risk to try crossing here. Could be better upstream, but that means going back to the fork to head uphill again. And we might have to go off the track.'

'Anything been sighted from the chopper?'

'Nothing. And they're losing visibility with this fog rolling in. They'll stand down any minute but will be available for air rescue if we need them for transport later.'

Adam had a vision of a small person strapped into a

basket stretcher being rushed to a big-city hospital with a high-level trauma centre. He shivered despite the warm coat he was wearing. As if she'd felt his discomfort, Sam swiftly turned her head.

'All good?' There was concern in her eyes.

'Yep.' Adam wasn't going to waste his breath on chatting. The sooner they got to where they could cross this damn creek, the better.

It was frustrating to have to go back the way they'd come to take another branch of the track that led further up to a lookout. Adam found himself taking a sideways glance at the woman walking just ahead of him. Even the profile of Samantha Gillespie's face indicated a keen intelligence. He guessed she was about his age, in her mid-thirties, given that she'd been working as a qualified general practitioner and then gone back to specialist postgraduate training in emergency medicine. She certainly seemed to know what she was doing and seemed more than comfortable in what was becoming rather a challenging environment. Her expression suggested that she wouldn't want to be anywhere else. Was she *enjoying* this, even?

A flash of something like anger came from nowhere at the thought, but this Dr Gillespie didn't have her only child in danger, did she? Was she even a parent?

'How on earth could this have happened?' he muttered aloud. 'Surely schools have to check the weather forecast before taking kids on excursions like this?'

Sam turned again. 'Our forecast today was for fine weather. What's probably happened is that a separate system has built up faster than expected somewhere else. A flash flood can be caused by rainfall that's a long way away. It might have been fine when they crossed the first time and it's caught them by surprise on the way back. Or it's taken them longer than they thought it would.'

She had an English accent, Adam noticed. In that initial panic he'd been fighting, he hadn't even been aware of that either.

'Hold up!'

The line of orange-clad searchers came to a sudden halt.

'I heard something,' Colin called.

Adam strained to hear anything other than the rumble and splash of fast water over big rocks they'd just left behind them.

'Yes…' Sam was nodding. 'I can hear it. A whistle.'

'Let's split up.' Colin was making some rapid adjustments to their plans. 'Some of us will go back to where the bridge was and the rest can go a bit further to hunt for another ford. Alec, you lead that group. Tom, you come back with us—you're our rope expert. If anyone *is* close to that point, we might have to make an attempt to cross. Sam, we'll need your medical skills. Adam— you come back with us, too. It's going to get a lot more rugged trying to follow the stream uphill and I intend to keep you safe.'

The beat of the helicopter rotors was directly above them when the news of hearing a whistle blast was shared and they were on their way back to where the bridge had been washed out. The downwash of air was a freezing wind but the radio message was enough to push them forward even faster.

'Target spotted,' Colin shouted as he got a direct message from the helicopter crew. 'Female adult. Came out to wave but had a nasty slip on the mud and only missed going into the water because she hit a rock. She was still mobile enough to crawl back into the trees so visual contact's been lost.'

It might well be Miss Kempsey, Adam thought. She would be desperate to alert rescuers to where she was keeping her pupils safe and she'd just had a sharp reminder that they needed to be far enough away from the muddy bank to not risk them slipping into the current.

This time, as they stood beside the remnants of the bridge, they could see the shadowy shapes of small people amongst the trees and ferns on the other side of the rushing water. They could also see someone lying on the ground in the midst of the huddle, a child sitting beside them. Adam couldn't be sure but…wasn't Charlotte the only one in her class that had long, dark braids like that? His heart rate sped up. He wanted to grab that remaining steel cable and drag himself across the creek without wasting another moment to find out how safe it might be.

Perhaps it was just as well that Colin and Tom were between Adam and the cable. So was Sam. Tom held onto the end that was still anchored on this side and lifted his feet off the ground. He bounced a couple of times.

'Seems solid,' he said. 'But there's no way of knowing what condition the other end's in.'

'I'm the lightest,' Sam said. 'What if I attach a rope to the cable with a carabiner and leave you guys with another rope clipped to my harness? That way, if the cable's not solid, I've got you for backup and I won't get swept too far downstream. If I get over, I can attach a backup rope on the other side and we can start getting these kids out.'

Adam had never realised before just how powerful

hope could be. He could see the frown on Colin's face and knew that what Sam was planning to do was still enough of a risk to give him pause as the group's leader. He picked up a stick and threw it into the water, presumably to gauge the speed and turbulence, and he was still frowning.

He watched Sam working with Tom to attach ropes and carabiners to both the cable and the harness she put on. With a big coil of orange rope over her shoulder, she lifted her chin to clip the buckle of a helmet and her gaze met Adam's for a heartbeat. He knew that she was very aware of the risk she was about to take. He also knew that it wasn't going to slow her down, let alone stop her.

Her courage was impressive enough to make him catch his breath and he felt as if he was holding it for as long as it took for Sam to pick her way through the torrent and then up the slippery mud on the other side. She went straight to the huddle of people in the trees. He saw her crouch to check the figure on the ground and then he saw her hold her arms out to gather one and then another child into her arms for a reassuring hug.

One of those children was crouched beside the adult figure and it was easy to recognise her as she turned and held her arms up for a hug, her braids swinging. Adam could actually feel that hug himself and it was the closest he'd been to tears since he'd got that alarming phone call about the danger that Charlotte might be in.

He held his breath, hoping that his daughter might be the first one chosen to be brought to safety, but she turned away from Sam, curling into the crouch she'd been in before, and it was another child that he watched being put into a harness and clipped to Sam for the return journey, their legs and arms wrapped around her like an oversized monkey. It felt as if everyone on this side of the roaring stream, including new police personnel arrivals and the returning members of the search and rescue group, was holding their breath now. With a child in her arms, the combined weight was a lot more strain on the intact cable and Sam took the crossing slowly and carefully, not wanting to slip and put a sudden, even greater, pressure on the lifeline.

Colin unclipped the child and carried him straight to Adam. The little boy was cold and frightened but didn't seem to be injured.

'*Mikey…*' Adam was not only his family's doctor, Mikey and Charlie were great friends. They'd gone through pre-school together and were now in the same class in primary school. 'Does anything hurt?' he asked. 'Did you fall over?'

Mikey shook his head.

'Can you take a really deep breath for me? Does that hurt?'

Another head shake.

'I'm going to wrap you up in one of these special shiny blankets.' Adam took a foil sheet from its package. 'You're going to be carried down the hill and back to school, where someone will be waiting to take you home. Your mummy always picks you up, doesn't she?'

Mikey nodded this time. 'This will help keep you warm until Mum can give you a big cuddle. Plus, you'll look like a Christmas present. Or maybe a baked potato?'

It was the first smile he'd seen, but then it wobbled. Mikey was looking up at the strangers looming over him as they could see Adam was finished with his primary survey.

'Where's my mummy?' he asked in a small voice.

'She'll be waiting for you,' Adam said. 'At school. This is Tom. He's going to find someone to take you down the hill so you can go and get that cuddle. Is that okay?'

Mikey's nod was uncertain but he let Tom pick him up. Adam turned his attention back to the stream where, already, Sam was making another crossing with another frightened child in her arms.

Not Charlotte.

None of the first four children were injured so all they needed was a quick triaging check from Adam, a foil blanket and someone to ferry them down to the transport waiting to get them home and warm. He was standing at the edge of the creek when Sam carried the fifth child over.

'Charlie's next,' she told him. 'She's fine. She just refused to leave Miss Kempsey. She's sitting there holding her hand.' She was smiling at Adam. 'She's a real sweetheart, your daughter.'

Oh, *man*…

Adam was so damn proud of Charlotte that the lump in his throat felt the size of one of those boulders in the stream. He had to clear it as he helped the child step out of the harness. 'How's the teacher?'

'She won't even let me look at her until all the children are safe. Said she's probably just sprained her ankle.'

It obviously took some persuasion to convince Charlotte to leave her teacher behind. Adam saw Sam pointing at him as she talked and he waved. Charlie waved back but he could see that she was still shaking her head. Then his radio crackled.

'Adam? Are you receiving?'

He pushed the talk button. 'Loud and clear.'

'Can you tell Charlie that she needs to come back to you so that I can look after Miss Kempsey?'

'Can she hear me?' He saw Sam holding her radio out to Charlotte. 'Charlie,' he said in his firm parental voice. 'You've done a great job looking after Miss Kempsey but you have to come back now, okay? Right now.'

'Okay, Daddy...' Charlotte stood up and stepped into the harness Sam was holding. She clung even more tightly than the other children had, with her face buried against Sam's shoulder so that she didn't have to look at the rushing water. Her face crumpled as soon as she saw her father and she was sobbing by the time he scooped her up but she wasn't injured. Adam wrapped her in foil and was holding her in his arms again when he got another call from Sam.

'Are you game to cross the stream?' she asked him. 'I could use some assistance over here.'

The other members of the team had heard the exchange on their radios. Colin and Tom were both staring at him, waiting for his response. Adam hadn't expected this. He'd imagined that he would be the one to carry Charlotte down the track, but he recognised the calm request for assistance that was covering something that Sam was seriously worried about.

'On my way,' he responded.

He took just another second to squeeze Charlotte. 'I have to go and help Miss Kempsey,' he said. 'So you need to be a brave girl and go back to school with one of the helpers here.'

'But... *Daddy...*'

'No buts.' Adam took her to one of the police officers

on scene. 'I've talked to Gamma and she's waiting for you at school.' The beat of gratitude that his mother was always there to help fill in any gaps in childcare was nothing new. It had been there from before his daughter had even been born—when they'd learned what the future held for them all.

'I'll see you very soon.' He pressed a kiss against Charlotte's dark hair and then turned to walk to where Tom was waiting, a rope coiled over his shoulder, holding out a harness for him.

It was ridiculous to feel this nervous, he thought a short time later as he held the two ropes that anchored him to the cable above him. How many times had Sam negotiated these slippery rocks and the push of rushing water to get across and back? Not only that, but she'd provided comfort to the children she'd been carrying—including his daughter—and she hadn't looked remotely as if she was as scared as he felt in this moment.

Adam took a deep breath. He could do this. He wanted to do this, and not just because Sam had asked for his professional assistance.

Maybe he wanted to impress Samantha Gillespie.

As much as she was impressing *him*?

CHAPTER TWO

Wow...

Sam hadn't been entirely sure that Adam would take up the challenge of getting across the stream. Especially when he'd finally managed to get his arms around his daughter again. It said a lot for his professionalism that he handed the little girl to someone else and turned back. She could see how nervous he was about the crossing, too. With good reason. The water—that was cold enough to feel like liquid ice—was flowing so fast it was impossible to see where a secure foothold might be, but Adam was clearly listening to the instructions being called by Colin and Tom that Sam could also hear faintly.

'Grip the rope with both hands. Chest height.'
'Face upstream.'
'Shuffle your feet across the bottom—don't lift them.'
'Keep low. Bend your knees.'

Adam was taking his time, both in the water and then on the slippery mud.

Then he was beside her, but he wasn't even looking at her and she didn't mind a bit. Because Adam's attention was focused on their patient and he had a smile on his smile that was so warm it was almost counteracting the chill that had got into her bones after a dozen journeys through the icy water of that stream.

'Hey,' was all he said.

Miriam Kempsey's jaw dropped and she took the mouthpiece out of the inhaler she was using for pain relief. 'You're Charlie's dad,' she said. 'What are *you* doing here?'

'First of all, I'm here to say thank you for looking after my daughter.'

The young teacher tried, and failed, to smile because her lips were wobbling. 'I think it was Charlie looking after *me*,' she said.

'Miriam's broken her ankle,' Sam said. 'But I can't splint it yet.' She moved the cover of one of the foil sheets she had opened to show Adam the very deformed ankle with the foot twisted into a horribly unnatural position, the skin stretched so tightly over the point of a broken bone that there was a high risk of it becoming an open fracture, with all the complications of infection that could follow. What was worse, the whole foot was ghostly pale.

'No pedal pulse,' Sam told Adam. 'Capillary refill greater than five seconds. Paraesthesia. No movement. Ten out of ten pain.'

Adam's attention was on Sam now. He was listening intently and she could see that he understood exactly what needed to be done before they could move Miriam without risking making this injury a whole lot worse. He also knew how urgent it was, given the disruption to both the blood supply and the nerves to her foot that this displacement had caused. He raised an eyebrow.

'What do you need me to do?' he asked. 'Get an IV line in? I'm guessing your hands are frozen.'

'Blocks of ice,' Sam had to admit. Doing something that needed fine muscle control like getting the tip of a needle into a vein was not going to be easy. 'Yes, if you can get a line in, that would be fantastic.' She handed him a zipped pouch that contained everything he needed to insert a cannula into a vein. 'The methoxyflurane is helping, but we need conscious sedation to reduce the fracture enough for splinting.'

'No worries.' Adam pulled on a pair of gloves. 'Can you hold your green whistle with one hand while I put a line in your other arm, Miss Kempsey?'

She sucked in another breath of the painkiller and then took the inhaler out of her mouth again. 'Call me Miriam,' she said.

Adam grinned. 'Not sure I can. Charlie adores you. We talk about you *all* the time at home, and you're never anything other than Miss Kempsey.'

Miriam managed the ghost of a smile this time. Adam glanced sideways at Sam, who was opening the drug pouch to draw up what they would need for the conscious sedation.

'You going to use a fentanyl/midazolam mix?'

'No. Ketamine.'

He turned back to his part of this task.

'Sharp scratch,' he warned Miriam. 'There we go… nearly done. We're going to get you out of here soon.'

'It's not going to hurt, is it?'

Adam was filling a syringe with some saline to flush the line and make sure it was patent. 'Sam's going to give you the good stuff any moment and we'll sort your ankle enough to be able to move you. You won't feel a thing. Even better, you won't remember it afterwards.'

Sam had her syringe full of the powerful drug that was going to make the procedure of shifting the bones in Miriam's ankle back to a position where they could be splinted to prevent ongoing or new damage to her foot as painless as possible. She was just waiting until Adam had secured the line with a plug and covered it with an adhesive dressing. For a general practitioner who probably didn't get to insert an IV line every day, he'd made it look easy.

He caught her gaze again as he smoothed down the clear, sticky covering, one eyebrow lifted, making it clear that she was in control here and he was ready to assist.

'Okay...here we go.' Sam attached the syringe to the plug. 'You might feel a bit weird in a few seconds, Miriam. Like you're floating.'

She was watching for the moment the drug took effect and it didn't take long. Miriam's eyes were wide open but unfocused—she was completely detached from what was happening around her. Her breathing and pulse were steady.

'Can you hold the top of her leg while I put some traction on?'

Adam circled the thigh with his hands, providing an anchor. Sam cradled Miriam's heel and foot in her hands and then began to apply pressure to pull and manoeuvre and align the bones.

Adam was watching Miriam carefully. 'You're okay,' he told her when she groaned. 'You're safe.'

'Where am I?'

'Where would you like to be?'

Oh... There was a note in his voice that Sam could feel right down to her bones. A lovely, masculine rumble and the hint of a promise that, whatever Miriam would like, he would do everything he could to make it possible.

'At school,' Miriam said slowly. 'Story time, on the mat…'

'Lovely,' Adam said. 'What story are you going to read to us?'

Sam didn't find out what the choice of story would be. She felt the pop of the dislocated joint going back into place and, within seconds, some colour began creeping back into the deathly pale foot.

'Good job.' There was approval in Adam's voice now and the praise was disconcertingly welcome.

'We've got a pedal pulse again,' she said briskly. 'Now we need to get this splinted well enough to get her to hospital for some X-rays. Can you grab the SAM splint from my kit, please?'

The effects of the drug were wearing off by the time Sam had wrapped the lightweight splint, made of soft aluminium strips inside layers of foam, around Miriam's ankle and bandaged it securely in place.

'Have you done it yet?' she asked. 'It doesn't hurt any more.'

'Can you wiggle your toes for me?'

There was movement. And a more normal capillary refill of just over two seconds.

'Can you feel me touching your foot here?'

'Yes.'

'That's really good.' Sam nodded. She was more than happy with what they'd achieved.

So was Adam. 'There's a stretcher coming our way right now,' he informed Miriam. 'It's got your name on it.'

More ropes had been strung across the stream while Sam and Adam had been working on stabilising Miriam for transport. The water level had dropped significantly since this rescue effort had begun and it was now much easier for other members of the team to bring a basket stretcher across. Well wrapped in foil blankets and strapped into the stretcher, Miriam looked snug and comfortable.

Adam helped Sam pack up her gear as a chain of people took the stretcher across the stream.

'Time to get our feet wet again,' he said, standing up with the larger medical pack in his hands.

Sam was about to protest and say she would carry her own pack but then he smiled at her.

'I owe you a big thank you,' he said. 'For getting my daughter across that torrent safely.' There was respect in his gaze. Admiration, even? 'I had no idea how cold and downright scary that was until I did it myself.'

Oh, *my*… What was it about this man's voice that reached places in Sam's body that shouldn't be accessible to a stranger?

And that *smile*…

Adam Carter wasn't simply ridiculously good-looking, he was quite clearly a very nice man as well.

Thank goodness it was time to follow her patient and look after her as she was transferred to her hospital and possibly sent on to a specialised orthopaedic team elsewhere. There was no time to think about whatever personal things were going on here.

That beat of attraction…a pure, physical pull that was strong enough to take her off-balance—if she allowed it to. Beat? Sam knew perfectly well it was actually more like the swirl of an impending tornado, but that only made it even more fortunate that she couldn't give it any head space. She wasn't going to allow herself to sink into that seductive pull. Why would she?

Her path hadn't crossed with Adam's in the whole time she'd been in this small town so far. It was unlikely that they would see each other again and, for heaven's sake… he had an adorable young daughter.

He probably had an equally adorable wife waiting for him at home.

Adam could not stop thinking about her.

Even amongst the relief of finally being at home and able to cuddle Charlotte, knowing how lucky they were that everything had ended as well as it did, he couldn't stop an errant thought of Sam Gillespie sneaking into his head.

He could see her, holding Charlotte just like this, wading through that icy, dangerous stream to bring her to safety.

And then Charlotte wriggled free and tugged on her father's hand to let him know that she was going to ask something very urgent.

'What's happened to Miss Kempsey, Daddy?'

'She hurt her ankle,' Adam told her. 'But Dr Sam looked after her so that it didn't hurt so much and all the people there helped carry her across the stream and down the track to where the ambulance was parked. We took her to the hospital for an X-ray and then a helicopter came to take her to a bigger hospital in case she needs an operation.'

Charlotte's eyes filled with tears. 'An *operation*?' Her voice wobbled. 'You mean she won't be at school tomorrow?'

'No, sorry, sweetheart. She definitely won't be at school tomorrow. She'll need some time at home too, when she gets out of hospital, and she'll be using crutches for a few weeks.' He wiped away the fat tear that had fallen. 'She said to tell you that she's going to be okay and she'll come and visit everyone at school just as soon as she can.'

But Adam was thinking of Sam again. Not only her confidence and skill in delivering medical care but her courage in being there on the rescue team in the first place and, even more so, volunteering to be the first to test the strength of that cable when the water was still at a high enough level to present a very real danger.

He'd never met a woman quite like her before. He couldn't deny that it was…intriguing, but it was also more than a little disconcerting. He hadn't felt a spark of interest in a woman to this degree since Charlotte's mother had died.

He'd never wanted to.

And that thought was more than enough to shut Samantha Gillespie out of his thoughts while he had a long, hot shower and then sat down to the very welcome hot dinner of roast chicken, crispy potatoes and homemade gravy that his mother had cooked for them.

'I thought this needed to be a bit of a celebration,' Jude Carter said. 'Thank goodness nobody got badly hurt.'

'Miss Kempsey did.' Charlotte hadn't picked up her fork. 'She's going to need clutches.'

Adam and Jude shared an amused glance.

'Crutches,' he corrected with a smile. 'But she's going to be okay, so try not to worry. I forgot to tell you that it made her feel so much better, the way you looked after her and held her hand while Dr Sam was busy rescuing all the other children. And you know what Dr Sam said?'

Charlotte shook her head.

'She said that you were a real sweetheart.'

'Aww…what a nice thing to say.' Jude was smiling at her granddaughter. 'And she's right, you *are* a sweetheart. Can you eat your dinner now, please? It's your favourite.' She glanced at Adam. 'Who is this Dr Sam? I've been hearing about her ever since Charlie got back to school. She sounds like some kind of superhero.'

'She works in the emergency department at Coromandel Hospital. She's new in town, I believe. I'd never met her before, but…'

He loaded his fork with a combination of meat and potato and gravy and felt a burst of anticipation at how delicious this mouthful was going to be. Or did that feeling have something to do with the fact that, yet again, he was thinking about Sam?

'I'm sure I'll see her again,' he said. 'I'm in that department sometimes.' He winked at Charlotte. 'I'll see if she's got a red cape hanging on a hook somewhere, shall I? Like that Supergirl dress-up costume you've got?'

He put his food in his mouth which made a natural end to that line of conversation, but he was still thinking about Sam and this time it was a much more personal memory.

He could see her eyes. They were hazel, weren't they? A golden sort of brown. What was more memorable, however, was that gleam of intelligence and more—a love of adventure? A love of life, perhaps?

Yeah…there was a glow about her, that was for sure. Something very, very attractive.

Despite himself, he knew that he *wanted* to see her again. Maybe he could drop into the emergency department some time tomorrow, just to follow up on what treatment Miriam Kempsey had ended up needing for her ankle.

* * *

Thursday turned out to be an exceptionally busy day at the Karaka Medical Centre so Adam didn't get a long enough break to walk down the hill to the hospital. He did, however, get time to ring his friend Jake who was a consultant emergency specialist there. They'd met not long ago, when Jake had brought his nephew, Arlo, in for an appointment and the possibility of potential friendship had been strong enough for them to arrange to meet up outside of their professional arenas.

'Adam…how are you? How's Charlie? I hope she wasn't too traumatised by what happened on her first school outing? I heard all about it this morning.'

'It was an adventure, all right. They've got a counsellor in to talk to the kids today, but the only thing that really bothered Charlie was that poor Miss Kempsey got hurt. I'm hoping to find out how she got on.' He hesitated only briefly. 'Is Sam around?'

'She is, but she's busy with a patient at the moment. Shall I give her your number and get her to call you back?'

'No, no, no…' Adam's knee-jerk response was a little over-the-top but, good grief…the last thing he wanted was for Sam to think he was desperate to speak to her in person. 'I just wanted to know if she ended up getting surgery on that ankle.'

'Apparently not,' Jake told him. 'Probably thanks to you guys doing such a good job on scene. Sam said she couldn't have reduced it without your assistance and it could well have become an open fracture if you hadn't been able to splint it as well as you did.' It sounded like Jake was grinning. 'She sounded pretty impressed with the way you went through that flooded river to help her.

Maybe you should join LandSAR too, and get the kind of excitement in your life that Sam can't live without.'

'I get plenty of excitement in my life,' Adam said. 'And you know as well as I do how impossible it is to commit to something that can be that time-consuming when you've got kids.' He hesitated again, but couldn't stop the query that was on the tip of his tongue. He could at least make it not too direct. 'I'm guessing that Sam either has a very accommodating husband or that they don't have any kids yet?'

'Mate…' Jake gave a huff of laughter. 'Husbands and kids are dirty words as far as Sam's concerned, although she did say that Charlie was totally adorable.' He chuckled again. 'I've never heard her mention a partner of any kind, but she hasn't been here that long. Might *not* be here that long either. She's clocking up some ED experience as part of her dream of getting a job in a rescue service. Are you sure you don't want me to give her your number?'

'*No.* I mean yes, I'm sure.' Did his tone give away the grimace on his face? 'Thanks, but I've got all the information I was hoping to get. Charlie's going to be very happy to hear that her darling Miss Kempsey didn't need an operation.' He needed to change the subject now. 'While I've got you, Mum's been saying it's time you and Isla and Arlo came round for dinner again. What's next week looking like for you guys?'

'Mmm… I love your mum's cooking. And Arlo loved teaching Charlie to play fetch with Ben. Let me talk to Isla and I'll get back to you.'

'No worries.'

Adam found himself smiling as he ended the call. He told himself it was because Miriam Kempsey was not as badly injured as they'd feared. It wasn't because Samantha Gillespie had been so impressed with his contribution to the callout yesterday.

Or the fact that she was single.

Not that it mattered. He didn't really go into the emergency department of Coromandel Hospital all that often. And Sam must have plenty of days off, anyway, so the odds of their paths crossing again any time soon were not high.

Given that she might not even be in town for that long made it possible that they'd never see each other again, in fact, and this totally unexpected level of interest he was experiencing meant that that was probably a very good thing.

CHAPTER THREE

THE INVITATION CAME out of the blue.

The junior department of the local primary school and their families and friends wanted the pleasure of Dr Samantha Gillespie's company on Friday afternoon so that she could be presented with stories and pictures that had been inspired by the dramatic turn of events at their recent school outing. The children would also be thrilled if she could tell them what it was like to be a doctor who went out on search and rescue adventures.

'You can't *not* go,' Jake told Sam when he saw the way she was shaking her head. 'Arlo told me about this. The whole school is allowed to go and see the display of stories and pictures from the juniors. He's really looking forward to it.'

'But I don't *do* kids,' Sam protested.

'Oh, come on… I've seen you working with anything from screaming babies to sulky teenagers. You're *great* with kids.'

'Not *en masse*.' Sam could feel her face scrunching into lines of something bordering on fear. 'What would I say to them? What if they ask weird existential questions and all their parents are standing around expecting me to be able to answer them?'

Oh, help…what if one *particular* parent was there?

When Sam was finally getting on top of pushing recurring images and sound bites of Adam Carter out of her conscious thoughts. She couldn't do anything about her dreams, mind you, but they would naturally fade, given a bit of time—like that sensation of butterflies having a party in her stomach had when she'd managed to stop thinking about the way he'd looked at her when he was thanking her for bringing his daughter to safety.

The rise of Jake's eyebrow gave her an alarming impression that he might be reading her thoughts.

'Adam tells me that his daughter is besotted by you. She's insisting on wearing her Supergirl costume every day, as soon as she gets out of her school uniform. She says she's playing being Dr Sam.'

Sam bit her lip. So Adam was being subjected to reminders about her on a daily basis? How embarrassing would it be to see him again? And to meet Charlotte's mother?

'He probably won't be able to make it,' Jake added. 'They're short-staffed at the medical centre this week with a bug that's going around. He's really disappointed because Charlie's teacher will be there and he wanted to know how she's getting on with that broken ankle. She's not back at work yet but she's making a special effort to hop there on her crutches.' Jake was giving Sam a stern look. 'Probably because she wants the chance to thank *you* in person and give a shout out to the whole LandSAR team. Wouldn't it be a great opportunity to encourage all those parents to make a donation to the service? Or to sign up some new volunteers?'

'Okay…' Sam's sigh was one of defeat. 'You can stop twisting my arm. I'll go.'

'Wear your rescue overalls.' Jake gave her a thumbs-up. 'And take a medical pack and a coil of rope to throw over your shoulder. They'll love that.'

Sam was walking away, shaking her head, but Jake wasn't finished. 'Oh, yeah…if you've got your red cape handy you could put that on as well. I'll tell Arlo to keep an eye out for you.'

It was actually quite fun.

The pictures and stories were really cute, with stick figure people and helicopters that looked very aerodynamically unsound and captions that had been dictated to a teacher and then signed with charmingly wobbly letters.

'Dr Sam took me over the river. I was really scared.'

'When we went to see the Kauri tree, the bridge got lost.'

'I was sad that Miss Kempsey hurt her foot.'

'Dr Sam was nice.'

'I hugged the Kauri tree. I hugged Dr Sam too.'

This last one was signed by Charlie and there were several large Xs. The headteacher told Sam that they would all be collected for her to take home later. There were smiling parents and proud children who gathered to sit on a mat at the front of the classroom where Miss Kempsey was sitting on a chair, her crutches leaning against the blackboard. There was an empty chair beside her.

'Please come and sit down, Dr Sam. We'd love to hear you talk to us about being a rescue doctor. The children have lots of questions.'

Sam sat on the tiny chair, her feet close to the first row of small children. The little girl right in front of her was Charlotte Carter. Parents were at the back of the circle, sitting on more of the child-sized chairs or standing in front of cupboards.

'Hi,' Sam said. 'Thank you so much for inviting me and I really love all your pictures and stories. You've put a lot of work into them.'

Several hands shot up in front of her. Miss Kempsey pointed at one of the children.

'Yes, Keiran?'

'Which one did you like the best?' Keiran asked.

'I like them *all*,' Sam said with complete sincerity. 'I couldn't possibly pick one that's the best.'

Other hands were waving but Miss Kempsey said she wanted to ask the next question.

'We were really scared,' she confessed. 'Weren't we, children?' She waited for the enthusiastic affirmative murmur and the smiles and nods from the parents to finish. 'So, we were wondering, were you a little bit scared too, Dr Sam?'

'Well…a little bit,' Sam agreed. 'But it wasn't just me there. There was a whole team of people who are specially trained so I knew they wouldn't let me do anything that wasn't safe. And I love being outside and doing things like going to rescue people.'

A little boy's hand shot up. 'Do you like helicopters?' he asked. '*I* do…'

'I *love* helicopters,' Sam said. 'And fast boats and abseiling down cliffs and…' she caught Miss Kempsey's expression and reined back her list of the potentially dangerous activities she favoured '…and I love being a doctor. That's my *real* job.'

Charlotte's hand was up now. 'My daddy's a doctor,' she said. 'And he was there helping too.'

'He certainly was,' Miss Kempsey said with a smile. 'And look…here he is now.'

Sam's heart skipped a beat and sped up noticeably as she shifted her gaze to the tall man coming into the classroom.

Miss Kempsey was beaming. 'Now we can say a proper thank you to both Charlie's dad *and* Dr Sam.'

She started clapping. The children and then the parents followed suit and Sam could feel her cheeks going pink. Adam was holding up his hands in a gesture of surrender but he was smiling, too. And then his gaze met Sam's and his smile faltered.

Could he feel it, too?

This…what *was* it? A shaft of sensation that was so strong it felt like a punch in her gut, but it wasn't unpleasant.

Oh, no…

It wasn't unpleasant *at* all.

The last question, from a little boy with wide eyes, was whether it was fun doing dangerous stuff, and he also wanted to know what the *most* dangerous thing was that Sam had ever done.

Both Miss Kempsey and the headteacher looked as if the school bell ringing at that point to mark the end of the day couldn't have been better timed. There were some more thank yous and more clapping and then a flurry of activity as pictures and stories were gathered off the wall for Sam to take home and the class collected their coats and bags and put chairs up on the tables.

All the adults whose children had been in the stranded group wanted a chance to thank Sam in person and she heard a lot about what an emotional day it had been for the families and how grateful they all were that it had ended as well as it did. Sam stood up to chat and shake hands but Miriam Kempsey was still sitting on the little chair nearby, talking to Adam, whose hand was being tightly held by Charlotte. She could hear snippets of their conversation and learned that the cast would be on her ankle for several weeks yet but she would be able to be back in the classroom as soon as she'd had another orthopaedic check and a moonboot fitted. She couldn't wait, apparently. She was missing her class. Judging by the bouncing from Charlotte, the children were missing her just as much.

The last person to come up to Sam was a woman with hair just starting to go grey and a lovely smile.

'I'm Charlie's grandma, Jude,' she said. 'I've been so excited at having the chance to say hi.' Her smile widened and the warmth in it made it obvious that she was Adam's mother. 'And to thank you. We'd really love to invite you to come and have dinner with us this evening. And you too, Miss Kempsey.'

Sam blinked. She didn't dare catch Adam's gaze.

'Please,' Charlotte begged. 'Please, please...*please*...'

'I'm afraid I'll have to say no,' Miriam said. 'I'm only supposed to be out for a little while today. I have to go home and put my foot up to rest now.'

Charlotte didn't let go of her father but she pulled him so that she could get hold of one of Sam's hands as well. '*You'll* still come, won't you, Dr Sam?' Her tone was a little desperate. 'Gamma's making our favourite special dinner just for you. It's roasty chicken.'

An abrupt silence fell. Adam broke it just before it got really awkward.

'You never know, Charlie,' he said. 'Dr Sam might be a vegetarian. She might not want to eat roasty chicken.'

Was he offering her a way out of this invitation? Because he didn't want her in his house? Sam couldn't quite interpret the mismatch of an amused gleam in his eyes with the serious tone of his voice, but she was taken aback to see Charlotte's eyes filling with tears.

'You're *not*, are you? A vegetable sort of person?'

'No.' Sam didn't want to be responsible for any tears. She smiled to be even more reassuring. 'I love roasty chicken. It's one of my favourite dinners, too.'

Charlotte was bouncing again. 'So you'll come? *Yay...*'

'Ah...' Sam hadn't had any intention of accepting what had been a totally unexpected invitation, but her gaze flicked up from Charlotte's beaming smile to catch one on her father's face. He knew exactly the predicament she was in. She held his gaze in a silent plea to help her out.

Oh, *my*...

Those *eyes*...

Sam Gillespie wanted something from him and what man could refuse a woman who looked at him like *that*? As if he was powerful and important enough to be able to help any damsel in distress. As if she had total faith in him and would be forever in his debt if he would do this for her. He had been as surprised as Sam at his mother's impulsive invitation to join them for a meal. If she was hoping for an escape route, he could easily defuse Charlotte's excitement and suggest another time might be better for the wonderful Dr Sam to come to dinner at their house. Another time that might never arrive because Sam didn't want to spend time with the Carter family. Or with him. Why would she?

And why on earth would he *want* her to?

He'd survived the most traumatic weeks—*months*, even—that any man could have gone through when he'd lost the mother of his child and become a single dad to a fragile, premature daughter. When the day finally came that he could take his tiny baby home and start a life he'd never imagined living, he was sure of only one thing. That he was going to be the best father he could possibly be to Charlotte. By default, in those early years it meant there was no time or interest in a life outside his work or the tight circle that was his family. He'd become comfortable being a single father. He'd never had the inclination to go looking for a relationship of any kind, which was why it had been such a shock to feel that flash of… interest…in Sam.

Okay…this totally unexpected level of physical attraction.

Acknowledging that, as part of the lightning-fast mental processing of how he felt about Sam being invited to dinner, led to a surprising conclusion.

Was it actually possible that Sam *might* want to come and spend some time with his family—and more specifically with *him*—because she was as aware of this unusual hum in the air between them as he was and she too was wondering what might be causing it? This thing that felt like a sound that was almost inaudible but he could feel it in his body like a kind of vibration—something he'd never felt before. Ever. This wasn't like any spark of physical attraction he'd experienced so far in his life. Was Sam as intrigued as he was?

But then again, perhaps it was because she didn't want to spend any more time with him. It was only a split second of eye contact but Adam could imagine that he was seeing something else in her eyes behind that plea. That she might know more about this hum than he did? That she knew exactly what kind of music it might turn into if it got louder? And that it might be…just a little bit dangerous?

Okay…that did it. He *had* to try and find out at least a hint of what it was—it was simply too compelling.

He held her gaze, mainly because he couldn't make himself break it. And he could feel his smile getting wider.

'*Please* come,' he said. 'It would make us all very happy.'

He saw the way Sam looked from Charlotte's hopeful face to his mother's smile. 'Are you sure?'

They could both see his mother and daughter nodding enthusiastically. Charlotte was doing that cute bouncing thing she did of going up and down onto her tippy toes.

'I'd say that's an affirmative from all of us,' he said. 'Mum's going to take Charlie home and I need to go back to the clinic for a while, but give me your address and I can pick you up on my way home later.' One eyebrow quirked. 'When you've had time to change out of your superhero gear.'

'No, give me *your* address.' Sam looked resigned to her fate now. 'I can walk, as long as you live in town.' She winked at Charlotte. 'Otherwise, I guess I might have to fly.' She smiled at Jude. 'What can I bring?'

'Just yourself,' Jude firmly. 'Charlie and I have everything sorted.'

CHAPTER FOUR

ADAM LIKED THAT she brought a chilled bottle of white wine with her, anyway. A favourite Pinot Gris of his, in fact.

Charlotte came to answer the doorbell with him, wearing her current favourite costume out of the dress-up box—the red skirt and the blue top with the diamond-shaped 'S' logo on the front and the red cape attached to the back.

It broke the ice very nicely.

'Wow,' Sam said. 'I finally get to meet a *real* super-hero.'

Charlotte giggled and then went suddenly shy, pressing herself against Adam's leg. He ruffled her hair. He felt a little shy himself, to be honest. They didn't often have a stunning-looking woman on their doorstep and Sam did look amazing in those faded skinny jeans tucked into black boots that made her legs look impossibly long and a close-fitting top under a cardigan that did nothing to hide her curves. Adam gestured to invite Sam into the house and realised that this was, in fact, the first time he'd ever brought a woman to the home he shared with his daughter.

Except he hadn't, had he? This wasn't remotely like a date. This was due to an invitation from his mother, not himself, and Sam had made it clear that she wanted to be independent and didn't want him to pick her up or take her home. This was simply Jude's way of thanking someone who had played a significant part in rescuing her precious granddaughter from what could have been a very sticky situation. Adam could feel that sudden tension evaporating as he let out a long breath.

'Come on through,' he invited, leading the way down the central hallway. 'We don't stand on ceremony around here. We tend to gather—and eat—in the kitchen.'

The kitchen was Adam's favourite room. It ran the width of the back of the house and had two sets of French windows opening into a big garden. The original coal range, set into an old fireplace, was only there now for its decorative purposes. His mother was closing the door of a very modern oven. She wiped her hands on her apron and came to greet Sam with a hug.

'I'm so glad you could come,' she said. 'We don't get visitors nearly often enough, do we, Charlie?'

Adam ignored the less than subtle reminder that there could be more to his life than his work and time at home with just his daughter for company. He held up the bottle of wine Sam had given him.

'Can I interest you in a glass of this excellent wine?' he asked. 'Did I tell you that it's one of my favourites?'

'Is it?' Sam's eyebrows rose. 'Mine too. I would have been a bit lost if I'd known dinner was going to be roast beef instead of roasty chicken because I know absolutely nothing about red wine. It gives me a headache so I never drink it.'

It was good to have a task to cover any hint of residual tension he was feeling but, as he found glasses and fossicked in a drawer in the hutch dresser for a corkscrew, he realised that he didn't need to worry. Charlotte had everything in hand. She showed Sam where she was going to sit at the table—right beside her.

'Do you like having a boy's name, like me?' she asked Sam.

'You know what?' Sam sat on her chair, which made her the same height as Charlotte. 'I really do. I love it when someone looks surprised because they expected me to *be* a boy.'

'Is it your real name or short for something? Charlie's short for Charlotte, but nobody calls me Charlotte.'

'Sam is short for Samantha. I never liked being called Samantha because it always sounded like I was in trouble. My mother and father refused to call me Sam.'

Was it an English thing to be so formal in referring to one's parents? Adam raised his eyebrows as he handed her a glass of wine. 'Were you in trouble often?'

'Sadly, yes.' She was smiling at him. 'But I grew out of it.'

Oh…that hum was distinctly louder as Adam wondered what sort of trouble Sam had got into when she was younger. He took a long sip of his wine, hoping that would wash the sensation away.

'What part of England did you grow up in?' he asked.

'London.'

'What's London?' Charlotte asked.

'One of the biggest cities in the world,' Adam told her. 'Way, way bigger than Auckland.'

'But Auckland's this big…' Charlotte threw her arms out wide. 'It's got a zoo, even. Gamma's going to take me there again. Aren't you, Gamma?'

'I am.' Jude was pouring gravy into a jug. 'I've got a

friend I need to visit and I thought Charlie could come with me for a weekend away.'

'Sounds fun,' Adam said. 'Am I invited too?'

'No.' Charlotte shook her head firmly. 'It's just us girls, isn't it, Gamma?'

'That's the plan.' Jude winked at Charlotte as she put the gravy jug on the table. 'I hope everybody's hungry tonight. Dinner's all ready.'

'I'm *starving*...'

Adam took another sip of his wine as he watched Charlotte push her chair a little closer to Sam's before she climbed onto it. So he was going to be left on his own for a weekend?

No. He wasn't going to allow his thoughts to go in the direction they'd suddenly spotted. It didn't matter if he had a weekend to himself. Or if Sam might be at all interested in something a lot closer to a date than a family dinner. It couldn't happen. This was a pinprick of a town compared to London and it was not possible to keep something discreet. Imagine if Charlotte heard that he'd been on a *date*? With someone she had put on a pedestal just as high as the one Miss Kempsey occupied that was only for people that were worthy of the greatest admiration and love. He remembered Charlotte's imminent tears at the idea that Sam might be a vegetarian. How much worse could it be if that pedestal got even higher? If she got the idea that...that...

It was very easy not to let that thought turn into words. He put his glass down and picked up the sharp knife to carve the chicken. He put a drumstick on Charlotte's plate—her favourite because she was allowed to pick it up in her fingers to eat it.

* * *

The elephant in the room wasn't getting any smaller.

Sam had seen the table set with only four places as soon as she'd entered the kitchen and it was soon obvious that Adam's mother was totally at home both cooking a meal here and eating at this table, but she couldn't ask where Charlotte's mother was, could she?

Maybe because the idea that a woman had walked away from both Adam and his gorgeous daughter was so unthinkable, she knew something terrible must have happened. Having no idea how recent that might have been meant that saying anything could be a painful reminder, but her curiosity was steadily rising. So was the impression that Charlotte was one of the happiest children she'd ever met. Sam couldn't pick up the slightest hint that this was a little girl who was missing her mummy.

In the end, it was Charlotte who solved the mystery, thanks to Adam starting a conversation about what had made Sam decide to come to New Zealand. She didn't tell him how desperate she'd been to get away from her upbringing. Or the parents that had never been that interested in having a child in the first place.

'I had this idea that it's one of the world's greatest places to find adventure on your doorstep,' she said. 'Which isn't so easy to do in a big city like London.' She wasn't about to tell them the kind of adventures she *had* found in her younger days. 'And that was why I decided to do GP training, so I wouldn't be on call too often and I could get away in the weekends and do exciting things like abseiling and kayaking and a bit of mountain climbing. You know, all those cool things you see on any platform that is enticing people to come here. What do they call it? The world's greatest playground?'

Adam was blinking at her. 'Yes… I remember you saying you'd been a GP up north. And now you've retrained in emergency medicine? General practice not exciting enough for you?'

Sam nodded but screwed up her nose as if it needed an apology. 'I blame helicopters,' she said. 'I went on a mountain rescue course with a friend and he had quite a nasty accident. There was room for me to go with him and the crew was okay with winching me up and taking us both back to the city.' She let out her breath in a sigh. 'That was it. I'd fallen in love. Found the career I want to be in for the rest of my life. I'm getting closer to earning my fellowship in the Australasian College for Emergency Medicine and then I can focus on pre-hospital and retrieval medicine.'

'Sounds like a lot of study,' Adam said.

Sam nodded. 'I love learning new things.'

Adam raised an eyebrow but his tone didn't hold any criticism. 'There's lots to learn in general practice, too,' he said. 'But you're right. It leaves plenty of time to have other things in your life. Like a family.' He smiled at Charlotte. 'I never wanted to be anything else. We had it all planned, Charlie's mum and me. We were going to have our own medical practice here in Thames where we both grew up and we'd find a house big enough for six kids.' His smile gave her the impression that he was amused. Or possibly relieved? 'We're complete opposites, aren't we?'

Had he and Charlotte's mum been childhood sweethearts? They'd had their future all mapped out to remain in their small hometown and live and work together as they raised their family. *Six* kids?

'Yeah…' Sam couldn't have agreed more. 'We are.'

'Daddy says I'm six kids all rolled into one,' Charlotte told her.

Sam was about to laugh and say she could see why, but Charlotte hadn't finished speaking yet.

'And that's a good thing,' she added. 'Because I'm not going to get any brothers or sisters. My mummy's dead. She didn't even get to see me because she was asleep when I was born and she never woke up.'

Sam shut her mouth with a snap. She had no words available now.

'She still loved you. Right from the moment she knew you were in her tummy.' Jude got up to collect the empty plates. 'How 'bout you go and put your jammies on and then you can come back and have some ice cream for dessert?'

'Can I help?' Sam offered, reaching for one of the serving dishes. 'That was such a delicious meal, thank you so much.'

'No, you're our guest of honour.' Jude added the dish to her pile. 'Please just sit and enjoy your wine. I've got some cream to whip for our dessert.' Her smile was a little too bright, as if she was trying to lighten the atmosphere. 'I've made a jam roly-poly in honour of you being English. I hope it's turned out okay—I haven't made one for about forty years.'

Sam let Adam top up her glass. She had to say *something* to acknowledge the tragic story that had been shared.

'I'm so sorry for your loss,' she said as he finished pouring the wine. She caught his gaze.

She opened her mouth, wanting to say something more than those totally inadequate words, but nothing came out. How could she tell him that she knew what it was like to lose the most significant person in your life? Had he held his wife in his arms as she'd taken her last breath, the way she had with Robbie?

Oh… For a heartbeat, Sam could almost feel it again. That desperation of hanging on, trying to stop the person you loved the most in the whole world being ripped out of your life. She could feel the sting of tears that she knew were not going to reach her eyes but it felt as if Adam had seen them anyway because he was holding her gaze and there was a question in his eyes that morphed into something that looked very like empathy.

It was simultaneously both comforting and disturbing. She hadn't actually shared anything really personal and yet it felt as if they'd just taken a step that considerably closed any distance between them.

Sam cleared her throat. She *had* to say something.

'Charlie's a real credit to you,' she managed. 'And your mum.'

'I'm very lucky to have Mum around,' Adam said. 'I could never have coped on my own.'

'That's not true,' Jude said, coming back to the table to put a flat dish onto a trivet. Curls of steam were coming from the sticky pudding it contained. 'I'm the lucky one—to have you both in *my* life.'

'It *is* true,' Adam said. 'Nicky wasn't just asleep when Charlie was born. She was in a coma. She'd had an aneurysm rupture when she was twenty-five weeks pregnant. She was brain dead but the decision was made to keep her on life support for long enough to give Charlie the best chance of survival. We were hoping for thirty weeks but ran into trouble with organ failure and cardio-vascular instability.'

The words were calmly clinical but Sam could hear the pain of things being left unspoken that had to have been an unimaginable emotional roller coaster. With someone on life support in intensive care, the visible deterioration in condition would have been inescapable. The decision of when to turn off that support had been taken from their hands, but there had been another life to consider and a Caesarean section to perform.

'Charlie was born at twenty-nine weeks,' Adam added quietly.

Sam's breath had caught in her throat. How had he coped with the two sides of that coin that fate had delivered? On one side, having to say a final goodbye to the woman he'd planned to spend the rest of his life with and, on the other, meeting his tiny, premature daughter who was just beginning her fight for life.

'She was in NICU for nearly three months,' Adam added. 'Mum kept me going. I reckon she spent as much time in the hospital as I did.'

Sam finally managed to take a new breath but she couldn't take her gaze away from Adam. He had her full respect for the way he'd picked his life up again in the wake of such a personal tragedy and created such a happy little family.

This house was so full of love.

It was everything she'd never had in her own childhood and the sudden pang of longing for what she'd missed out on was unexpected. Painful, even. Did it show on her face? If it did, Sam could only hope that Adam would assume it was due to sympathy. His smile was certainly poignant enough to be acknowledging that.

'So I *am* the lucky one,' he said. 'Thanks to Mum, and being a GP with consistent hours and almost no on-call work, I've got the best life I could have wished for. I've got…' His smile lit up and he held his arms out as Charlotte hurtled back into the kitchen, now dressed in pink pyjamas but with her Supergirl cape still tied around her neck. '*You*,' Adam finished, wrapping his daughter in his arms. 'That's what I've got.'

The rain started while they were eating their jam roly-poly with whipped cream and hokey pokey ice cream. It was even worse by the time the dishes had been done and Charlotte was in the bathroom cleaning her teeth.

'Listen to that rain,' Jude exclaimed. 'It's cats and dogs out there. You can't walk home in this, Sam.'

'Maybe you could drop Sam off on your way home?' Adam suggested.

'I would, but I've promised to do Charlie's bedtime story tonight. We're on the last chapter of *Charlotte's Web*. If you drop Sam home you won't have to be part of all the crying that's bound to happen.'

'Sounds like a deal.'

Sam nodded. 'Our whole class cried their eyes out when our teacher read that chapter.' She gave Jude a hug. 'Thanks again. I think you're the world's best grandma.'

Charlotte wanted a hug, too. 'Will you come back next time we're having roasty chicken?'

'It was so good, I just might.'

They made a run for the car a short time after that, but Sam had water dripping from her hair as she climbed into the passenger seat. When Adam leaned towards her to click his safety belt buckle into place he could see that she had droplets of water on her eyelashes.

How cute was that? He had a ridiculous urge to put his fingertip close enough to catch the droplet when she blinked. Hastily, he turned to start the car.

'Sorry 'bout that.'

'What, the weather?' Sam laughed. 'Yes, I hold you entirely responsible for the heaviness of this rain.'

Adam pushed the damp spikes of his hair back from his face so he could see clearly to back out of the driveway onto the road. 'I meant how heavy it got inside. I thought someone at the hospital might have filled you in on our sad story, but maybe more than five years is long ago enough that people are forgetting. It's not as though the real drama happened here, apart from when Nicky collapsed. We were Auckland based for the best ICU and NICU facilities that were available. Now...' The change of tone was intended to signal an end to that topic of conversation. 'Where are we heading?'

'Burke Street.'

'Near the old wharf?'

'Yes. I found an apartment that's half an old house and a bit rundown, but I was sold on the idea of being able to run on that walkway every morning and watch the sunrise lighting up the sea and the land on the other side of the firth. It's the best ever way to start a day.'

Adam made a huff of sound. 'Sounds idyllic. I'm usually filling a lunchbox and making peanut butter toast and trying to get Charlie out of bed and dressed and then finding where she left her shoes last night and trying to braid her hair when I seem to have more thumbs than fingers.

The chaos only dies down after I drop her off at Mum's and get to work.' He glanced sideways with a smile. 'I'm not complaining. For me, it's a way to start my day that makes everything worthwhile.'

Adam stopped opposite the old house Sam pointed out and cut the engine. Sam unclipped her safety belt and reached for the door latch, but Adam touched her arm.

'Wait a sec. Give the rain a chance to slow down a bit or you're going to be completely soaked before you even get to your gate.'

They could hear the heavy rain drumming on the roof of the car in the silence that suddenly fell as Sam turned and caught Adam's gaze. They were between streetlamps here and the light was masked by the pouring rain anyway, so it was dark inside this small space. Not so dark that he couldn't see Sam's face, though, or feel the intensity of their eye contact. The question that had been haunting him couldn't be left unasked.

'Can you feel that?'

It looked as though she knew exactly what he was talking about and it had nothing to do with the beat of rain that was echoing in his body. This was the fizzing of some kind of chemical reaction. An attraction that was off the scale already, but somehow it was managing to increase.

'Yes...' The word was no more than a whisper. 'Absolutely.'

Perhaps a new element had just been added to the alchemy that was happening here. It wasn't simply the level of attraction; it was knowing that it was mutual.

And here they were. In almost darkness, behind a curtain of rain that made them invisible. Two adults who were seriously attracted to each other and there was nothing to stop them taking a step closer to where it might lead them.

Okay, Adam had a daughter who was the centre of his world and he would protect her with his life, but did that mean he had to walk away from a private moment that he might want purely for himself that nobody else would ever need to know about? Something that could never hurt Charlotte?

The rain seemed to be turning into hail and the sound of it hitting the roof was deafening. Sam wasn't going anywhere just yet and she seemed to be finding it just as difficult to break the eye contact as he was. A whole conversation was taking place in the fraction of time before either of them needed to blink.

I want to kiss you.

I want you to...

Just a kiss, that's all.

That's all we need.

Yes...that's all we need.

Adam loosened his safety belt so he could lean closer. He cupped Sam's chin in his hand and then his lips were on hers. Finally, the tension that had been escalating like the last moments of a bomb ticking was released.

It should have been enough. The touch of their lips. Sinking into a dance of pressure that was sending delicious tingles right through Adam's body. Who parted their lips first? Whose tongue joined the dance first? Adam had *no* idea and he didn't care. Nothing mattered except this kiss.

This *incredible* kiss...

He couldn't have said who pulled away first either, but it was clear they both needed some oxygen and they were breathing fast enough for the windows to be getting foggy.

Sam was staring at him. 'There's something you should know,' she said.

'What's that?'

'I don't do relationships.' Her voice was even, she was merely stating facts. 'I don't do kids. And I'm not going to be in town for long.'

The boundaries were very clear. That kiss wasn't going to be the start of anything. Adam found himself letting his breath out in a sigh of relief.

'I don't do relationships either,' he said. If the idea had ever occurred to him in the last five years it would have been dismissed so fast it might as well never have existed. 'But I definitely do kids.'

Charlotte was his world. His life.

He could feel his lips curling into a smile that might have a poignant edge to it. 'Just as well, isn't it? It could never have worked, given that we're such complete opposites.' He leaned in and pressed another, brief kiss to Sam's lips. 'There's something wild about you,' he murmured. 'I'm not surprised Charlie thinks you really are a superhero. See you around, Sam.'

'Thanks for tonight.' Sam took no notice of the rain as she got out of the car. She threw a grin over her shoulder. 'Great kiss, by the way.'

The door slammed shut. Sam darted across the road and vanished behind a gate.

So that was that.

But Adam Carter was smiling. All the way home.

CHAPTER FIVE

THE PLATOON OF TALL wooden poles that had once held up the Burke Street Wharf were dark shadows as the sky behind them showed the first glimmers of daylight.

It was chilly and Sam was only wearing thin leggings and a matching sports bra that left her midriff and arms completely bare but she wasn't feeling the cold as she did her warmup prior to starting her run.

She was buzzing.

She'd got back to Thames late last night after being in Auckland for an intensive four-day course on pre-hospital retrieval medicine and it had been the most exciting few days she'd had in decades. This was the light at the end of a long tunnel of hard work and study.

She went into a lunge, twisting her body towards her forward leg to activate her core muscles and then stretched her arms above her head as she stood up before repeating with her other leg.

How good was this? Being at the point where she could begin learning the practical skills she would need to bring to her dream career? Sam had soaked up every minute of the classroom time and, even better, actually doing things like the winch training from the platform in the huge hangar and practising safety around helicopters by staying low, avoiding the tail rotor, keeping all gear below head height and always remaining within the pilot's field of sight.

She was jogging on the spot now, lifting her knees to loosen up her hip flexors, and then she began running. Into the sunrise, watching the glints as the slightly choppy water of the sea inlet began to catch the light. She'd told Adam that this was the best ever way to start a day and today was no exception.

Mind you…the best ever way to *finish* a day had to be the way Adam had kissed her not long after she'd told him about these morning runs. She'd thought about that kiss more than once in the last few days. A lot more than once, in fact—partly because the picture Charlotte had drawn of 'Doctor Sam' was secured to her fridge with magnets so she saw it every time she opened the door. The taller stick figure had a red smudge that was clearly the cape of a superhero, which made Sam smile every time she looked at it. The reminder that the artist's father had given her the best kiss she'd ever had gave her smiles a secret edge that she suspected was adding considerably to her current satisfaction with life.

That saying about opposites attracting wasn't wrong, was it?

The last few days had confirmed that Sam could never go back to being a family doctor like Adam. She'd been there, done that, and it had been stifling. General practice was a completely different planet to the one she was earning her passport to, with its edge of danger and the excitement of not knowing what challenges the next job would bring. That night with Adam's family had also reminded her of why she was choosing to never get into a committed relationship or even think of having children.

They were both anchors that would have held her back and made it impossible to be doing exactly what she wanted to be doing with her life.

It wasn't simply that Adam was happy in a job as a GP that she'd found so restrictive and yeah…a bit boring. The reminder of why she avoided having people that close to her had been much sharper. Her heart had bled a little, remembering what it had been like to hold someone who meant everything to you and watch their life slip away. It had been bad enough doing that with her best friend. It would be unthinkable to do it with someone you'd chosen to spend the rest of your life with. Or, possibly even worse, with your own child?

That was definitely something that Sam was never going to risk having to experience.

Her feet hit the ground in a steady rhythm and Sam was feeling weightless, almost as if she was floating, and part of this feeling of freedom came from the knowledge that her choices meant she *was* free. The world was her oyster and she was within touching distance of the pearl she wanted the most. She could go anywhere, any time without any constraints. She was single. Childless. She didn't even have a pot plant that required regular watering.

Sam checked her watch and slowed down enough to turn and head back home to have a quick shower and then head in to start her shift in the emergency department of Coromandel Hospital. She increased her speed, pumping her arms.

Yep…she was definitely on the right track in life. She could no more go back to being a GP than give up her freedom and career by saddling herself with family responsibilities—however happy Adam Carter appeared to be with his life.

Not that she was about to forget him as she ran forward into her exciting future. Oh, no…nobody would ever forget a kiss like that.

Had Adam been thinking about it in the last few days?

Had it occurred to him that one of the things they had in common was that they were on exactly the same page when it came to relationships, even if he had no idea that it might be for similar reasons?

That they liked the same wine?

And that, judging by that kiss, they were both clearly very attracted to each other?

Sam stopped by the old wharf again, this time to bend over, with her hands on her knees to catch her breath.

Also judging by that kiss, sex with Adam Carter was quite likely to be off the charts in terms of how good a physical encounter could be. So good, Sam found herself thinking, as she stepped under the hot water of her shower a few minutes later, that it might be regrettable not to experience it. Rude, even?

Just once.

A one-off, absolutely no-strings kind of thing.

How good would *that* be? Not that an opportunity was likely to present itself, given the mix of shift work, a small child and the need to avoid fuelling any small-town rumour mill, but…there was no harm in simply thinking about it, was there?

It had been a long day.

Adam had left home early to add a commute time of over an hour to get to Hamilton and attend an endorsed advanced cardiac life support workshop to maintain his certification as part of his continuing professional development. He didn't mind doing it, because while it was fortunate that he didn't often get the chance to put his skills in CPR and airway management to the test, it was all too easy for those skills to get rusty and undermine the confidence to use them when they were essential.

And things were always changing. Adam was thinking about the astonishing advances in laryngeal mask airways as he drove home again that afternoon. Some models had video technology now, to aid with placement and safety, others had drainage channels and chambers to protect against aspiration, and it was even possible to intubate through an LMA now. It was high time that Adam updated what he carried in his first aid kit, he decided. He might even splash out on one of the fancy ones that could be used as a bridge to the secure airway that intubation would provide. The list of advantages for the device had been impressive—being able to change to a tracheal tube without losing oxygenation levels, being able to avoid neck extension in suspected spinal injuries—

The rest of the list evaporated from his head as Adam got closer to the intersection where the road that led to the east coast of the Coromandel Peninsula joined the highway he was on. His foot moved to the brake of his vehicle as he tried to make sense of what he was seeing at the roundabout ahead of him.

A fully laden logging truck was coming down from the challenging road through the hills that was the main route to the east coast. Fast. Was it due to the weight of the huge vehicle and its load? Had something gone wrong with the brakes? It certainly wasn't slowing down as it approached the roundabout. A small red hatchback was ahead of it, taking a right turn to head towards Kopu or Thames. A delivery van was about to enter the roundabout heading in Adam's direction and the silver SUV in front of him had stopped to give way to the truck that should, in fact, have been slowing to give way to the van. Instead, the truck seemed to be gathering speed and the trailer full of logs was rocking. As it barrelled into the roundabout, clearly out of control, massive tree trunk logs broke one of the chains holding them onto the truck's trailer and some logs bounced onto the road, one of them crushing the roof of the van on the other side of the roundabout. The cab of the truck then clipped the waiting SUV, which tipped and rolled sideways, finally landing on its wheels with its chassis badly dented and airbags deployed. As the SUV was rolling, the truck trailer jack-knifed and tipped, taking the cab with it, skidding sideways to block two of the roundabout's entry and exit points, including the one in front of Adam.

For a stunned moment, he simply took in the horrific accident site. Then he flicked his car's hazard lights on to warn anyone coming up the road behind him and opened his door to get out. In the wake of the cacophony of the shocking crashing and banging of the collisions and the screech of brakes and metal on metal, the blaring of the single horn of the badly dented SUV was the only thing to break an ominous silence. He could smell diesel and petrol and the burnt rubber on the road from the failed attempt to stop the truck. What Adam couldn't hear—or see—was any sound or movement from the passengers of any of the vehicles involved.

He had his phone in his hand and he was scanning the scene as he activated an emergency call.

'Emergency. What service do you require? Police, fire or ambulance?'

'Probably all of them,' Adam responded. 'I'm at the intersection of the Kopu-Hikuai Road and Ngati Maru Highway. Logging truck vs two smaller vehicles.'

He rapidly answered more questions as he began walking into the scene. No, he didn't know how many people were involved yet. Yes, there were hazards. He couldn't get close enough to see if the driver of the truck was alive because there was no way of knowing how stable the logs were. He couldn't see the driver of the van beneath its crumpled roof and broken windscreen and all he could see of the SUV so far was someone slumped in the driver's seat. Police were going to be needed to control traffic that was already starting to arrive from three directions and the fire service would be needed to deal with the logs and any extrication that was required.

He had to stop providing information in order to direct people who were getting out of their vehicles now and approaching the roundabout.

'Stay back,' he warned. 'Some of these logs could roll.'

He shouted to others to move their cars to the side of the road to leave room for emergency vehicles to get through. He could already hear a siren in the distance as he walked swiftly towards the SUV, which seemed well enough away from any loose logs to be safe to approach.

'Help…' The driver was trying to open the door now but her call ended in a sob. 'Please…my little boy's in the back.'

Adam tried the door but it was jammed shut.

'Help's coming,' Adam shouted. 'Are you hurt?' He

could see a trickle of blood on the woman's face. 'Are you having any trouble breathing?'

'I… I don't think so. But Jamie… *Ah…*!' The woman cried out in pain as she twisted to try and undo her safety belt. 'My arm… I've hurt my arm… I think it might be broken.'

'Try and stay still.' Adam could hear a child crying. He shaded his eyes to see past the glare of the sun on tinted windows and saw a boy who looked about three years old, strapped into a car seat that looked reassuringly undamaged. The crying meant he was conscious and his airway was open and Adam could also see small arms and legs moving. He tried to open the door but it was almost as jammed as the front door and only opened an inch or two.

'Jamie? Can you hear me?'

'Mummy…' The wail was terrified. '*Mummy…*'

'It's okay, Jamie,' Adam called. He had to go and check the other vehicles in this first, rapid triage. 'We're going to get you and Mummy out very soon. I'll be back in a minute.'

He ran to the van next. The passenger side of the vehicle had been completely crushed by the log that had then rolled onto the road and was now some distance away. The driver's seat had been knocked flat and a young man was lying on it, still in his safety belt, his eyes open but his face looking very pale and frightened. The door was half open, which let Adam feel for a pulse as he spoke to the driver.

'My name's Adam. I'm a doctor. Emergency services are on the way.' He could feel a radial pulse, which told him that the young man's blood pressure was adequate for the moment but the heart rate was rapid. So was his breathing.

'My *legs*,' he groaned. 'I can't move them…'

The log that had come down on the roof had pushed the dash down far enough to trap the driver's legs. Not just trap them either. Adam could see that it was compressing both legs enough to be a real problem.

'What's your name?'

'Jason.'

'Are you having any trouble breathing, Jason?'

'No…it's just my legs…' His groan was agonised. '*Help me…*'

'You're doing really well, Jason.' Adam could hear more than one siren now. 'Focus on your breathing. I'll be right back.'

The first vehicle was a fire engine, coming past a line of cars on the other side of the road. Right behind that was an ambulance. Adam walked to meet them and pass on the limited information he'd gathered so far. To his astonishment, the back doors of the ambulance were thrown open and Samantha Gillespie jumped out. She had a high viz vest on over her scrubs and a backpack kit in her hands.

'*Adam*.' She looked horrified. 'Oh, my God, were you involved in this accident? You're not hurt, are you?'

For the tiniest blink of time, Adam registered how good it felt that she was concerned for him, but it was gone and forgotten just as quickly.

'First on the scene, that's all. What are you doing here?'

It was one of the paramedic crew who answered, as he came from the driver's seat. 'The call came when we were in ED so Sam decided to jump on board.'

Of course she had. Adam wouldn't have expected anything else.

'Hey, Liam.' Adam knew the local ambulance crews. They sometimes transported patients to the medical centre if they needed help but weren't unwell enough to go to the emergency department or were called to pick up someone with chest pain perhaps who *was* unwell enough to be there.

'I've only triaged,' he told them. 'Three patients who are all conscious. There's a young mum and a child trapped in the SUV that rolled about three times after it was clipped. I couldn't get to the truck's driver. The cab's under all those logs. The guy in the van is the priority. He's got his legs trapped under the dash with enough pressure to be causing a crush injury. His airway and breathing are okay but he's in severe pain.'

Liam reached into the back for another trauma kit. 'Looks like the firies are assessing the stability of that pile of pick-up sticks. We might be able to check the cab soon.'

Police cars were arriving now, traffic was being controlled, a scene command vehicle had just parked and fire crews were setting up gear like stabilising chocks and hydraulic cutting tools.

'Where do you want to be first, Sam?' Liam asked.

'I'll go to the guy in the van,' Sam said. 'Adam's right to be giving him priority unless you find the condition of anyone else has deteriorated. Can you go to the woman and child in the car? Let the scene commander know what we're doing and yell if you need either me or Adam to assist.'

She was already moving as she looked over her shoulder at Adam. 'Come with me?' she asked. 'We'll get started but I might have to leave you to carry on if they can get access to the truck cab for me to see what's going on with that driver.'

At least he didn't have to wade through a raging river to assist Sam this time, Adam thought. He flicked a quick text message off to his mother to let her know that she might need to stay later with Charlotte after school and then glanced behind him at the mess of the giant spilt logs. He could imagine Sam scrambling over them to get into the cab as soon as she could, but right now she had a laser focus on what was waiting for them at the van.

Jason looked even paler than he had a few minutes ago. His airway, breathing and circulation were all still within acceptable parameters but his pain, if anything, was worse. Sam had to squeeze into the small space of the half-open door, working on someone who was lying awkwardly on a seat where the back had been knocked flat, but she was making it look as normal as if she did this sort of thing every day as she slid the beam of a penlight torch into each of his eyes to check his pupil reactions. Adam had the same feeling as he'd had on that first day he'd met her, but he didn't think it was anything like an enjoyment of a potentially catastrophic situation this time. He could feel that she was simply in her element—doing what she was born to do, even? She was impressive, that was for sure. Calm, controlled and *so* focused. The tone of her voice was reassuringly confident as she talked to Jason, letting down the pressure on the cuff around his arm after getting a blood pressure reading.

'What would you give the pain on a scale of zero to ten, with zero being no pain at all and ten the worst you can imagine?'

Jason swore succinctly. '*Twenty…*' he groaned.

'I hear you.' Sam was unrolling a drug kit. 'I'm going to give you something right away to take care of that pain for you.'

'*Please…*' Jason begged. 'Do it fast. Knock me out.'

Sam wriggled backwards far enough to get some kits out of her backpack. She handed one to Adam.

'Can you find me a three-mil syringe and an MAD in this IV kit, please?'

'MAD?' Adam wasn't familiar with the acronym.

'A mucosal atomisation device. Small pack like an IV cannula. It's got a soft foam-tipped nozzle and a Luer-lock connector.' Sam was unrolling a drug kit. 'I'm going to give Jason some intranasal fentanyl to get on top of his pain fast.'

A fire officer came to stand behind them as Sam was administering half the dose of the drug into each of Jason's nostrils.

'You'll feel the effect of this in just a few minutes,' she told him. 'Hang in there, buddy. You're doing really well.' She looked up at the fire officer. 'I'd like to get him out of here as soon as we can, but it's going to need to be a very controlled extrication, especially when it comes to taking the weight off his legs.'

How long had it been since Adam had used any of his knowledge about crush injury syndrome and the dangers of releasing the intracellular toxins that could build up even in the space of thirty minutes or so? The flood of myoglobin and potassium could cause tissue death from rhabdomyolysis, renal failure and even cardiac arrest and death.

Looking behind him, he could see that the two paramedics on scene were beside the SUV, the doors of which were being wrenched open with a crowbar. They had a stretcher beside them with equipment on it.

'Do you want me to get the defibrillator?' he asked Sam. 'ECG monitoring for any signs of hyperkalaemia?'

'Yes. Please.' The look she gave Adam was one of approval. 'I think we might be more in need of it. Another ambulance should be here soon and I'm going to make a call to see if there's helicopter backup available to get Jason transported.'

He heard her voice behind him as he turned away. 'See if you can find out anything about the truck driver, too.'

He did, but the news wasn't good. Adam shook his head as he carried the defib back to Sam. The firies were setting up their gear to cut the door off the van and create better access. 'Status zero for the truck driver,' he told her, letting her know that the man had not survived. 'It's possible it was a medical event that caused the accident.'

Jason was much happier as his pain score tracked down but Sam was moving with a controlled urgency, still in the cramped space between the door and the flattened front seat. She was relying on Adam to pass her everything she needed.

'Alcohol wipe, fourteen-gauge cannula, Luer plug and a clear dressing, please. And can you set up a giving set and bag of saline? I want to get fluids running as our first priority.'

Adam understood why. Fluid loading was top of the list in management of a crush injury because it could dilute the effects of any toxins that might be released. A patent IV line could also let them provide a medication like ketamine that would allow the greater level of pain relief likely to be needed during the extrication process.

The next minutes passed in a blur of activity and noise. Orders were being shouted and engines were running in the background to get heavy equipment in place ready to shift the logs that were blocking two main highways. A tow truck had arrived and was waiting on the sidelines for the go-ahead to move the SUV. Adam saw a policewoman holding the little boy from that vehicle, who looked much happier now, clutching a soft toy as Liam's crew partner was checking him for any sign of injury. His mother was in the back of the ambulance having her forearm and wrist splinted.

The loudest noise was coming from the hydraulic gear that was being set up and tested right beside them, but Sam seemed to be blocking out any distractions as she worked to get IV access on Jason's arm. Adam flushed any bubbles out of the line and handed her the end of the tubing, holding the bag of saline up to keep the line running after she'd attached it. Then he watched her swiftly sticking electrodes onto the young driver's chest and watching the screen of the defibrillator intently as it settled into providing a basic rhythm strip.

'We'll do a twelve-lead as soon as we're out of here,' she said to Adam. 'That will pick up the earliest signs of too much potassium, but I want to be able to watch for peaked T-waves or widening QRS complexes and especially for any arrhythmias or a sudden drop in blood pressure when we take the weight off his legs. Can you get some of the extra drugs we might need drawn up, please? We'll give him some sodium bicarbonate before we start the extrication but we could need insulin, calcium gluconate, salbutamol—'

'Are you guys able to step back for a bit?' A fire officer interrupted Sam's list. 'We need to cut the door off and then get the spreaders in between the footwell and the bottom of the dash so we can roll it up—and out.' He saw Sam's expression. 'We don't do that until you're ready and we can go as slow as you need.'

But Sam clearly had more on her mind than controlling the release of pressure in case of complications. She looked at the mangled passenger side of the van, shook her head and then leaned in, over Jason, to peer towards the back of the vehicle.

'Can you get the back door open for me? That way, I can stay close to Jason and look after him but not be in the way while you're doing the cutting. I don't want to leave him alone in there.'

Adam could see how concerned she was for her patient. He could imagine how noisy and scary it would be for this young man to be lying alone in a vehicle that was being cut up around him and the movement could easily cause a huge increase in pain which would only make it worse.

He could see just how much Sam cared and it gave him an odd lurch in his chest. For a moment, he almost envied any patient that had this woman looking after them. She not only had the skills and the courage to be able to do whatever needed to be done medically, she also had a level of compassion that gave those abilities a depth that was an absolute gift.

She was an astonishingly compelling person.

'What can I do?' he asked.

'Bring the kit around the back. I'll take the defib in

with me and hook it up again, but it'd be great if I can rely on you to draw up any drugs I might need or chuck me any other supplies.'

It only needed a crowbar to get the back door open and a few boxes hauled out to make room and Sam climbed inside without hesitation. Adam handed her the defib and went back to shift the rest of their gear out of the way of the fire officers as they moved in to stabilise the van, with blankets to protect Jason from any debris, and started using the 'Jaws of Life' tools of cutters and spreaders. He could see Sam inside the back of the van amongst some remaining boxes, crouched close to Jason's head as she helped hold the protective blanket above him.

He took a deep breath as the noise level increased, with the hiss and roar of the hydraulic tools and the pumps, the crunch and pop of metal being snapped, people shouting and, to top it off, a helicopter coming in to land just up the road. He could actually feel the beat of the aircraft's rotors in his body and then he could feel the van rocking beside him, presumably as supporting structures were broken and pulled away. Not that Adam moved an inch. He wasn't going anywhere.

Sam wanted to rely on him and he wasn't about to let her down. He liked being the person she could rely on. It felt surprisingly good, in fact.

To be honest, it made him feel a whole lot taller. Not as invincible as their local superhero, Samantha Gillespie, of course, but it did feel as if he was, temporarily at least, sharing a tiny patch of her adrenaline-soaked planet.

CHAPTER SIX

THE BEST FISH and chip shop in Thames just happened to be on the route that Sam took on her way home from the hospital.

When it was late enough to be dark and she'd had a long shift in the emergency department, the treat of an iconic takeaway meal that needed no effort whatsoever was too much to resist—especially when this shop took the food to a level that any chef might be proud to serve.

Sam ordered the gurnard fillet in tempura batter with a side of wasabi mayo and then, because she only indulged herself like this so rarely, she also ordered the truffle parmesan fries. She paid for her order and, as she moved to sit down on the row of empty chairs while she waited for it to be cooked, the bell over the door jangled as another customer came in.

Adam Carter.

She hadn't seen him since the accident, which was a few days ago now, so it took her by surprise how good it was to see him again. It also made her realise that she'd been thinking about him more than she had acknowledged during that period of time. Working so closely with Adam at the scene of that major accident had been very different to having him assist her with the management of Miriam Kempsey's broken ankle on the day of the flash flood.

This had been full-on, life-threatening trauma management—the kind of situation that made any lack of communication or understanding or discrepancies in skill levels between colleagues very obvious. Sam had found it easy to work with him the first time, but when they were both looking after Jason she'd been aware of an ease that usually only happened with someone you'd been working with long enough to have complete trust in them. Maybe that was what was continuing to surprise her when she thought back on that day—this professional connection that was in sync enough to confirm there was something unusual in their personal rapport as well.

Something that went above and beyond the undeniably unusual level of physical attraction?

Yeah…it was a little disturbing just how good it was to see him again so unexpectedly right now.

Adam hadn't noticed her because he went straight to the counter.

'You're about to close, aren't you?' His tone was apologetic. 'Have you got time for a last order? I got stuck doing some paperwork at the clinic but I've been thinking about your fish and chips for the last hour or more.'

The man behind the counter laughed. 'Anything for you, Doc. What do you fancy?'

Adam was staring up at the blackboard menu on the wall. 'What do you recommend today?'

'Try the gurnard in tempura batter.' Sam couldn't resist the opportunity to surprise Adam as much as he'd surprised her. 'Or the line-caught red cod.'

His head swung around and Sam loved the way his face lit up at the sight of her.

'Great minds think alike,' he said with a grin. He

turned back. 'I'll have what she's having.' He lowered his voice to a stage whisper. 'She's smarter than me.'

He came and sat beside her moments later. Right beside her, even though it was late enough for them to be the only customers in the shop and there was a whole row of seats. Small plastic seats. Small enough for Adam's thigh to be touching hers.

Sam sucked in a breath. 'Bit late for you to be out hunting and gathering, isn't it? And you were doing paperwork on a Saturday evening?'

'I know. Sad, isn't it?' But Adam was smiling. 'That's what you get when I'm left to my own devices. Mum took Charlie up to Auckland today. They've been to the zoo and out to dinner and now they're tucked up in their motel. They're going to have lunch with Mum's friend tomorrow. She *was* going to take Charlie to Rainbow's End in the morning, but there's been a change of plan.'

'Rainbow's End? That's the enormous theme park, isn't it? I've never been there.'

'It's got New Zealand's only roller coaster with a vertical loop and double corkscrew.' Adam shook his head. 'But apparently that excitement can't compete with the lure of red pandas and meerkats. Charlie's fallen in love and just wants to go back to the zoo.'

'Aw…that's cute. Is Jude upset that she's going to miss out on the roller coaster?'

Adam tilted his head and lowered his voice, as if he were imparting a secret. 'I think she's fallen in love with the red pandas, too.'

Sam laughed. 'So you've been left to your own devices and you chose to catch up on paperwork?'

'I've had my excitement for the week. That crash scene the other day was quite something, wasn't it?'

'It was. You're very lucky you weren't a few seconds further along the road. You could have been right on the roundabout yourself.'

'I know.' Adam's tone was suddenly sombre. 'When I had time to let it sink in later, it was definitely one of those reminders of just how fragile life is.' He cleared his throat in the beat of silence that was Sam's agreement. 'Not that we need any reminders of that in our line of work.'

'No.' Sam lowered her voice, even though there was nobody close enough to be hearing their conversation. 'Did you get told the results of the autopsy on the truck driver?'

'No.'

'Massive MI. He could have been struggling with severe chest pain as he came down the hill and dead by the time the truck tipped over.'

'What about Jason?'

'Apart from that badly fractured femur that needed a rod and external fixation, he's doing well apparently. Severe bruising and he's still got paresthesia from nerve compression, but that should heal. I spoke to one of the guys on the chopper crew later who said they monitored for any signs of crush injury syndrome but the only real issue was keeping on top of his pain relief.'

One of Adam's eyebrows lifted. 'Those guys were impressed with your pre-hospital management. I got the impression they're hoping you apply for a job on their base.'

Sam let her breath out in a huff of laughter. 'They're nice guys. And they know me now, thanks to a course I just did in retrieval medicine in Auckland. Angus was one of the instructors. They also know it was a team effort. You were great.'

She could see that their meals were almost ready. The wire baskets of deep-fried food had been lifted from the vats and the excess oil was being shaken off. A steaming heap of shoestring fries was being drizzled with truffle oil and then dusted with parmesan cheese. Sam's stomach rumbled.

'That smells *so* good.'

'Mmm...'

Adam's thigh grazed hers as he got to his feet and Sam jumped at the electric tingle it created. She found he hadn't moved as she stood up and they were suddenly even closer together. When her gaze collided with his, the tingle intensified so sharply the anticipation of her delicious dinner paled into insignificance.

And then it hit her.

There was no reason for Adam to go home to eat his meal alone, was there? It was oddly difficult to catch her breath. Not unlike how she felt at the end of a particularly energetic run when she had to put her hands on her knees to help haul in the oxygen she needed. Like she had been doing that day when she'd started thinking about how good sex with Adam Carter might be. So good that it might be regrettable not to experience it?

Just once?

Had the thought occurred to Adam, like it just had for herself, that this was not only the first opportunity they had for some discreet time alone together but that it could be the only opportunity they might ever have?

She was about to find out.

Somehow, Sam managed to keep her tone casual as

she broke that eye contact and headed for the counter to pick up the white paper-wrapped package of hot food.

'Why don't you come to my place to eat?' She threw a smile back at Adam. 'That way, your fish and chips won't get so cold.'

It became very clear, almost the moment Adam walked through Sam's front door and heard it click shut behind him, that this food might get stone cold before it got remotely near being eaten.

Then he turned, realising that Sam hadn't moved, even to turn on a light. She was leaning against that door.

Watching him.

Waiting for him to make the first move?

He'd known what he was doing when he'd accepted her invitation to bring his takeaway dinner to her place. He'd known exactly what this opportunity to be alone in this unexpected—and reassuringly discreet—encounter was going to lead to. The attraction had been simmering in the background ever since he'd met Sam. The heat had been turned up with that kiss as they sheltered from the rain that night and maybe it had been the click of that door shutting them off from the rest of the world that made it boil over. Adam could almost hear it sizzling as it met the flames.

So he made the first move.

He put the warm, steamy paper packages he'd been holding so that Sam could find her keys and open the door on the small table under the coat hooks, confident that when he turned, Sam would still be watching.

She was. And he caught the hint of approval in the subtle movement of her lips. He'd seen this woman in complete control of more than one situation now, but Adam knew instinctively that Sam didn't want to be in control in this moment. She wanted to let herself go and sink into the escalating fizz of sensation that was gathering around them. Hanging in the air. He could almost taste the effervescence as he sucked in a breath. He put his hands on the door on either side of Sam's head and, slowly, he leaned in to cover her lips with his own.

He heard the tiny sound she made.

How could so much be communicated in a sound that wasn't even close to a word?

It held a note of relief.

Pleasure.

Need.

A promise that this was all it would be. A moment in time. A gift—for both of them, but it didn't have a ribbon. There were no strings of any description attached to this. It was the kiss in the car all over again except that it wasn't going to stop until one of them wanted it to, and that sure as hell wasn't right now.

Adam had never felt a desire like this. This was the oasis in a desert he'd been living in for years. A physical release he'd started to believe he no longer needed. How wrong had he been?

Sam tried to lift her arms to put them around his neck but his body was so close they were trapped, so she slipped her hands around his waist instead and pushed them inside the back of his jeans. It was Adam's turn to groan as he felt her fingers burning the skin of his buttocks and pulling him closer to her own hips. He had to lift his mouth from hers to catch a breath and she tipped her head to the side, her eyes closed. He kissed the side of her neck and he could feel the way her pulse was racing. His hands were moving, finding their way to the hem of the top Sam was wearing, and she lifted her arms so he could peel it off. Then her hands were on him again, fumbling with the snap button and then the zip of his jeans.

Really?

Were they not even going to try and find the bedroom?

Apparently not.

Sam broke their kiss with a sound that was a word this time.

'Now… Right *now*… I can't wait…'

'But…'

'It's safe,' Sam whispered. 'I promise. I would never take risks.' She was breathless now. 'I *want* you, Adam…'

He believed her. And, dear Lord, he wanted *her*. He'd never wanted anything this much in his life. Sex that was… wild…that was what it was. Standing in a tiny, dark hallway with only the support of a door as they scrambled to shift clothing—just enough. Sam, with her arms around his neck, her face buried against his shoulder as he lifted her just far enough. With her back against the door and him supporting her weight, she lifted her legs further and wrapped them around him so tightly he couldn't tell where her body finished and his began. The cry of sheer ecstasy they both made a very short time later also mingled into one sound and then faded into the rasp of them both trying, and failing, to slow their breathing as they untangled themselves.

It could have been awkward. A 'What the hell have we just done?' kind of moment as they stared at each other.

But then Sam smiled and took Adam's hand.

'Come with me.' Her voice was husky. Dead sexy. 'I know somewhere a lot more comfortable.'

She didn't turn the lights on in her bedroom either. Adam followed her example and shed every item of clothing he was wearing and slid under the duvet with her but he still had the odd sense that Sam didn't want to be controlling this. This time, however, Adam had far more control over the flood of desire—or had it been raw need?

This time, he was going to make love to Sam. Slowly. He was going to find out exactly what turned her on and drive her crazy with anticipation. And then he was going to deliver and hopefully give her the kind of pleasure she'd given him with the gift of discovering an intensity to a physical act that he hadn't known even existed.

Perhaps it was because it had been too long since he'd had this kind of release.

Or, and Adam had to admit that this was quite likely, he'd never been with anyone like Sam. Both he and Nicky had lost their virginity together as teenagers and had never wanted to be with anyone else. Even the idea of a sexual relationship had not been of any interest since he'd lost Nicky, so he'd only ever known what sex was like with the gentle, loving soul that his wife had been.

If the sex in his past life had been the warm embers of a slow fire, there were flames flickering amongst those embers with Sam.

This time, he would deliberately slow things down so that the desire was a softer glow. Would those flames erupt again?

Oh… Adam really hoped so. He wanted that magic of those dancing shapes and the spikes of scorching heat along with the comforting warmth of where they were coming from.

* * *

It was well after midnight by the time the fish and chips finally got reheated in the oven.

Sam put the battered fish fillets on a plate, the crispy, cheesy fries in a bowl, grabbed a roll of paper kitchen towels and took them back to her bedroom. Adam was obediently sitting, propped against her pillows, having been firmly instructed not to move. Sam put the plates in the middle of the bed and sat cross-legged on the end, well covered now in an oversized tee shirt and soft leggings.

'I am *so* hungry,' she said, reaching for a hot chip. 'What did you do to me, Adam Carter?'

'I think it was more what *you* did to me,' Adam countered, but he was smiling as he picked up a piece of the fish. 'Don't get me wrong—I'm not complaining, here.'

Sam had her mouth too full to respond but she nodded agreement.

She wasn't complaining either. She'd been confident that sex with Adam would be off-the-charts amazing but it was fair to say that it had exceeded her expectations by quite a long way.

Who knew that a contented, almost country GP and single dad who was devoted to bringing up his child—not to mention his mother being still a huge part of his life— was hiding such an astonishing sexual prowess—along with an ability to understand non-verbal language that was impressive and a generosity that was heartwarming?

Sam knew now. And she was still smiling inside at the revelation. Best sex ever.

Too good, even?

Because it was enough to make her want more? A lot more?

No. That was enough to set off an alarm. She swallowed her mouthful.

'Well…at least we got that out of our systems,' she said. 'Normal service can resume.' Her glance was more serious than her tone. 'I was being quite sincere telling you it was safe. I have regular testing for any communicable diseases like HIV, have never had an STI and I have an IUD which provides more than ninety-nine percent effective contraception.'

Adam had also swallowed his food. 'I had the feeling that you wouldn't leave something that important to anyone else,' he said. One side of his mouth curled up. 'You're an intriguing mix,' he told her. 'Absolutely in control on the one hand and totally wild on the other.'

Sam grinned at him. 'It's called balance,' she said. 'Is the fish good?'

'Fabulous. That sauce is about as hot as you are, though. Beware.'

Sam hid her smile as she broke a piece of fish off and dipped it into the wasabi mayo. So Adam thought she was hot?

She liked that.

'Have you always been this wild?' he asked after they'd eaten in silence for a minute.

'Way wilder,' she confessed. She flicked him a glance that was screened by her well-rumpled hair. 'You have *no* idea.'

'Tell me.'

It sounded almost like a command. Or was it genuine interest? Sam had never told anyone about her past. But then, she'd never eaten fish and chips in bed with a man she'd just spent several hours getting to know extremely well.

'Have you heard of parkour?' she asked. 'Or freerunning?'

Adam was shaking his head.

'How 'bout roofing? Roof topping?'

'None of the above.'

'Have you seen videos of people who are mad enough to go running across rooftops and jumping from building to building? Running up a brick wall and doing a back flip off it? Or climbing skyscrapers or enormous cranes and then hanging by one hand or doing some crazy pose to take photos at the top?'

Adam had been looking increasingly appalled as she spoke. '*You* did stuff like that?'

Sam nodded. 'I know. It was stupid. Illegal and far too dangerous.' She let her breath out in a sigh. 'But I was young. And it was also very, very exciting.'

'But…' Adam was looking puzzled now. '*Why?* Why would you take risks like that? How old were you?'

'About sixteen.' Sam shrugged. 'Maybe I wanted my parents to notice I was missing. Maybe I thought that if I proved I was brave enough, someone would notice me. Or maybe I didn't think it would matter if I fell off the planet because nobody really cared. Except for Robbie. He was my best mate—the one who got me into it in the first place.'

'What made you stop?' There was a flash of alarm on his face. 'You *have* stopped, haven't you?'

Sam nodded. 'I only did it for a while.' She bit her lip. 'Got pretty good at it, though.'

'I can imagine.' Adam's tone was dry. 'What made you stop?'

'I got arrested.' The words probably shocked her as much as Adam. Nobody knew this about her. She wasn't intending to add to that confession but other, never spoken, words just tumbled out as well. 'And Robbie missed his jump.'

The silence said it all.

'You were there?' The question was quiet.

'Yeah…'

Sam finally looked up when Adam didn't say anything in response. She was intending to break the heavy atmosphere by saying something cheesy like that was when she'd decided to become a doctor so she could help other people who, for whatever reason, felt the need to do stupid things, but the words evaporated when she found his gaze on her.

She could see the empathy there and it took her back to that moment when she'd been sitting at his kitchen table and it felt as if he'd guessed the connection that felt like such a significant bond between them.

It wasn't simply empathetic. Adam's steady gaze suggested that he understood how guilty she'd felt that they'd been doing something stupidly dangerous, but there was no judgement there. It felt as if he'd put his arms around her. And then he *did* put his arms around her. He pushed the plates of food aside and took her into his arms and then leaned back against the pillows with her head on his chest. He didn't say anything. He just stroked her hair.

And Sam fell a little bit in love with him for that.

CHAPTER SEVEN

THE RHYTHM AND routines of a busy general practice were familiar enough to be a second home to Adam and by late Monday afternoon he was more than happy with what had been a busy start of another week as part of one of the key services that gave the community a safe place to live.

'You're looking very happy today, Adam.' Erin, one of the practice nurses, went past him as he came out of the office. 'Did you not get the memo that it's only Monday?' She gave him another glance as she continued on her way to the reception area. 'Or was it a particularly good weekend?'

Oh, *man*…

Now that he'd seen his final patient for the afternoon all it took to push open the mental door that had been kept firmly shut during working hours was an internal sigh of relief. Thank goodness nobody knew just how good it really *had* been. Nobody other than himself and Sam Gillespie knew that and nobody ever would. It was going to stay private. They'd both agreed on that.

'*This was a one-off*,' Sam had reminded him as he slipped discreetly out of her house in the wee hours. '*I don't do relationships, remember?*'

'*Neither do I. Getting a night to myself like this only happens once in a blue moon, anyway. It's all good.*'

Was it that good, though? As he remembered his words, Adam heard an echo of that old proverb in the back of his mind—that if something seemed too good to be true, it probably was.

Did he need to remind himself of why he couldn't get any closer? That he couldn't allow himself to fall in love with any woman because it wouldn't be only himself that would suffer if something happened. The risk of loss was always there, wasn't it? Not by death, necessarily, but it wasn't uncommon for relationships to not work out and that might be just as hurtful for Charlotte.

It was easy to shrug the thought away. No, he didn't need a reminder. It wasn't going to be a problem because he wouldn't allow it to be. Maybe there would be some kind of price to pay down the line but he'd make sure he was the only one out of pocket.

And that gave him permission to go back to that afterglow for a moment longer. To remember what else Sam had said.

'It's better than good. I like being proved right.'

Adam had stopped for a beat. Long enough to hold her gaze and let the heat build again—just a little—because it felt so good. His curiosity got the better of him, however. *'What were you right about?'*

'That it was as good as I thought it would be.'

Adam wanted to smile again now but, knowing that he might be revealing more than he had any intention of making public, he shrugged instead. He also kept his tone admirably neutral.

'Charlie certainly reckons it was the best weekend ever,' he told Erin as he caught up with her. 'Mum took her to Auckland Zoo—*twice*—and now she's started a campaign to get a red panda as a pet. When I said it would be against the law, she said she was going to write a letter to the Prime Minister to ask for permission. And that she would remember to say please, so he'll probably say it's okay.'

'I think your daughter must be the cutest kid in Thames,' Erin said. 'I hope you're going to make it happen for her.'

Adam laughed. 'Mum bought her a soft toy version in the zoo shop. I said I'd get her a collar and lead for it and she could take it for walks.'

'Adam?' The receptionist, Liz, looked relieved when she saw him. 'Would you have time to see Janet Morrison? She's come in without an appointment and everyone else has still got patients to see.'

'Yes, of course.' Adam followed her glance and frowned slightly when he saw Janet Morrison sitting underneath a poster advertising the healthy food pyramid. She smiled at him and he relaxed a little. Whatever it was that had brought her into the clinic well before her prescription needed a refill didn't seem to be distressing her too much.

'Come on through, Mrs Morrison,' he invited. 'You've come just at the right time.'

It really wasn't a problem if he had to stay later than usual to see Janet. As usual, his mum was doing the after school pickup and childcare and she was more than likely to have dinner ready by the time he got home.

As he led the way down the corridor and then held the door of the consulting room open, he found his mind drifting again—just for the few seconds it took for Janet to catch up with him—and now that that door had been pushed open there was only one direction his thoughts wanted to go in since that memorable night on Saturday.

Even the joy of having Charlie back home yesterday, brimming with the excitement of her 'girls' weekend' away with Gamma, hadn't been enough to keep them completely in line. He had, no doubt, made it worse by postponing sleep last night, reliving every minute of his time with Sam as he lay in the solitude of his bedroom, because he'd found he was still thinking about it during the morning chaos of making and eating breakfast, filling the lunchbox, finding Charlie's Mary Jane shoes and a clean school uniform polo shirt and getting them both out of the house in time.

It wasn't that he was thinking about nothing but sex. Oh, no... There had been a lot more to think about than that, no matter how mind-blowing it had been, but he hadn't realised quite how much until Charlie had arrived home and run to him for a cuddle. He'd held his daughter in his arms, basking in the warm glow of how much he loved her, and that was the moment that realisation hit him suddenly, that it was the last thing he'd expected to come across.

That he'd felt something eerily similar the night before.

When he'd been holding Sam in his arms after she'd told him about the wild escapades of her teenage years. Not that it was the wildness that had captured him on such a deep level. No...it had been what she had hinted at. That she'd been that reckless because she felt unnoticed. Unimportant.

Unloved, even...?

And then she'd had to watch her best mate die. She hadn't needed to tell him how harrowing that must have been. He could feel it, right down to his bones.

A chunk of his heart had broken off at the thought of

what she'd had to cope with before she'd even reached adulthood as he held this astonishing woman close to him. This incredibly clever, courageous, *caring* woman.

He had no room in his life for any kind of relationship and Sam didn't do them anyway, but that didn't seem to be an obstacle for a physical attraction suddenly becoming something very different.

Was he in danger of falling in love with Sam?

Was he simply feeling more alive than he had in years because he'd broken through the barrier that had kept him celibate for far too long?

Or was he beginning to realise how big the gap in his life might be and dreaming a little of what it might be like if it was filled?

Whatever. This wasn't the time or place to be thinking about it. And what was the point, anyway? It wasn't going anywhere, was it?

Adam was watching the slightly awkward way Janet seated herself in the chair beside his desk

'Is something hurting, Mrs Morrison?'

'Just my wrist,' she said. 'I think I might have bumped it on something in the garden today and given myself a bit of a bruise.'

Yes. That was why she looked as if keeping her balance was a bit of a challenge as she sat down. She was supporting her right arm with her left, across her chest— the kind of protective self-splinting that was indicative of something a lot more painful than he would expect a bruised or sprained joint to be.

'Let's have a look.'

Adam pulled back the sleeve of the elderly woman's cardigan to find himself staring at a swollen wrist, misshapen into the classic 'dinner fork' shape of a Colles' fracture. Even a gentle palpation of the bones in her forearm was enough to make her wince and, when he lifted his gaze, Janet Morrison was watching his face. She knew perfectly well that this was more serious than she'd suggested.

'Did you have a fall, Mrs Morrison?'

Her gaze slid sideways. 'What makes you say that, Dr Carter?'

He touched the end of her fingers. 'Can you feel that?'

'Yes.'

'Can you wiggle your fingers?'

The attempt was feeble.

'It's a bit sore, isn't it?'

She still wasn't meeting his gaze. 'A bit.'

He checked her capillary refill, pressing on the base of a fingernail and watching how long it took for the colour to come back to the cuticle.

'You're going to need an X-ray, Mrs Morrison, but I'm pretty sure you've broken your wrist. This looks very much like an injury which we call a FOOSH injury—a fall onto an outstretched hand. I'm going to find a splint so we can make you a bit more comfortable.'

He put a rolled-up crepe bandage for support beneath the palm of Janet's hand in the gap caused by the angle her wrist was frozen in and then used another to bandage the splint against her forearm.

'Can you tell me how it happened?' he asked. 'Were you really out in the garden?'

'Yes. I was planting all my summer pansies.'

'Can you remember what happened? Or did you just find yourself on the ground?'

'I can remember it perfectly well.' His patient sounded offended. 'I stood up and felt a little bit dizzy and when I tried to take a step I…must have tripped on something.'

Adam reached for the blood pressure cuff on the wall beside the chair. 'I'm going to give you a quick check and then call an ambulance to take you to the hospital for an X-ray. Would you like me to call your daughter so she can come to the hospital? She lives in Hamilton, doesn't she, so it might take her a while to get here.'

'Please don't call Claire.' There was a tremor in Mrs Morrison's voice. 'I don't want her to know.'

Adam was silent as he took her blood pressure. It was a little low, which could explain the dizziness. He listened to her heart and then finally asked what had to be asked. 'Is there a reason why you don't want your daughter to know about this?'

She nodded. 'It's because… I know what happens when you start falling over. Before you know it, they've put you in a home and…and…'

Tears were imminent. Adam took hold of Janet's un-injured hand.

'You're not about to be whisked away anywhere that you don't want to go,' he reassured her. 'What we do need to do is look after you and make sure that you're safe.'

The elderly woman was clinging to his hand and Adam dismissed his plan to call an ambulance to take her to the hospital.

'How 'bout I drive you up the road,' he suggested, 'and come in with you while they do an X-ray? If it's a straightforward break, it will only need a plaster cast on it and I can have a chat with your daughter while that's happening.'

'But you need to get home to your wee girl.'

'My mum's looking after her,' Adam said. 'I wouldn't cope without her in my life, and that makes me appreciate mums in general. I'm quite sure your daughter will want to be here with you as soon as she can but, for the moment, I can take her place.' He smiled at Janet. 'Because that's what I'd want someone to do for *my* mum.'

'Oh…' A tear or two slid from Janet's eyes. 'You're such a lovely young man, Adam. You so deserve to find happiness again after your troubles.' She accepted the tissue Adam passed her and wiped her eyes. 'And how wonderful would it be for dear little Charlotte to have a mother?'

Adam shook his head. 'Let me help you up, Mrs Morrison. My car's not far away.'

From the corner of her eye, Sam saw the moment when Adam came into the emergency department, a frail-looking elderly woman with a sling hanging onto his arm for support.

Jake was moving to greet them but there was no chance for Sam to say hi because an X-ray had just come up on screen and it was sending a chill down her spine.

She'd had a feeling that there was more to five-year-old Mikey's sore throat and difficulty swallowing than a cold or even something more serious like flu or RSV, but this was making the hairs on the back of her neck prickle. It was a side-on image of the neck and there it was—the distinctive 'thumbprint' of an enlarged epiglottis.

Jake was walking past her now with Adam and the elderly woman, but his steps slowed as he was caught by what was on the screen.

'Look at that, Adam.' Jake signalled a nearby nurse. 'Jess, could you please take Mrs Morrison here through to Orthopaedics? Suspected Colles' fracture. We'll catch up with her soon.'

Sam caught Adam's gaze, and caught that frisson of connection that should have been too personal to be professional but was also too powerful not to enhance any way they chose to connect.

'Epiglottitis?'

'Five-year-old boy. Michael Cameron. Came in with a fever, sore throat and dribbling a bit. Very anxious. So's his mother. He was one of the kids we rescued from that flooded creek.'

'Mikey?' Sam could see the way the level of concern in Adam's face deepened instantly. 'He's Charlie's best friend at school. Also one of my patients.'

'He remembered me from when I went to visit them at school for the thank you. So did his mum, Lou.'

Jake was nodding. 'It helped. Come and talk to them, Adam. Another familiar face. We need to do as much as we can to dial down the anxiety so it doesn't exacerbate airway compromise. If he gets really upset it could trigger a respiratory arrest.'

Lou was relieved to see them coming back into the room. 'I can't get him to keep the oxygen mask on his face,' she said. 'He keeps pushing it away.'

Sam could hear a new sound in Mikey's breathing that hadn't been there a minute or two ago. A high-pitched whistling noise that was being caused by air trying to get through airways that were becoming too narrow.

'Stridor's new,' she said quietly. The paediatric oxygen saturation clip in the shape of a green crocodile was still in place on Mikey's finger and a glance at the monitor showed her that the level of oxygen in his blood had dropped to only ninety-two percent.

Too low. The little boy was showing signs of struggling to breathe as well. He was leaning forward in the classic 'tripod' position and Sam could see accessory muscle use in the way his head was bobbing and his shoulders lifting. She caught Jake's gaze.

'We need a line in and fluids up and we need to secure his airway.'

'I'll page Anaesthetics. I might get some transport on the way, too.'

It only needed a single nod of agreement on Sam's part. They didn't have a paediatric intensive care unit in this hospital and she had a horrible feeling that little Mikey might be in need of one very soon. She could actually feel the tension ramping up as if it was another solid presence in this space.

Adam was perched on the side of the bed, doing a good job of distracting Mikey.

'So red pandas are really cute. They kind of look like little foxes and they're black underneath and red on top, but their ears and cheeks and nose are all white.'

'We'll have to go there soon, won't we, Mikey?' The brightness in Lou's voice was clearly an effort. 'It's been ages since we've been to the zoo. I don't think I've ever seen a *red* panda.'

Adam looked up as Sam pulled an airway trolley closer to the table. She also opened one drawer and then another on the IV trolley, putting items onto the top.

'We're going to get Mikey to breathe in a medication

that will make him sleepy enough for me to be able to get a line into a vein in his hand,' she explained to Lou.

'Where the cream is?'

'Yes. That's helping to numb the skin, but we don't want to frighten him so being sleepy and relaxed is important, too.'

It took only a short time for the anaesthetic gas to have the desired effect. Sam put a tourniquet around Mikey's arm and swabbed the back of his hand. 'Can you steady the hand for me while you're there, please, Adam?'

'Sure.'

Sam carefully edged a small cannula into the vein and then secured it with a sticky cover and a bandage to protect the Luer plug from being bumped. Jake was setting up the IV fluids and a nurse was holding an oxygen mask close to Mikey's face when it happened.

The little boy made a strangled sound and then stopped breathing.

Adam jumped off the bed and helped Sam flatten the end and then tilt Mikey's head back to try and open the airway. Lou stepped back, her hand over her mouth and her eyes wide and terrified. Adam had his hand on her arm as Jake handed Sam a laryngoscope.

'I can't see a thing,' she said, seconds later. 'There's too much swelling.'

'Surgical airway kit?' Jake was by the trolley.

Sam glanced at the monitor. Oxygen levels were dropping rapidly. 'Let's start with a PTJV,' she said. 'I want to get the oxygen levels up.'

Percutaneous transtracheal jet ventilation was an emergency procedure using a needle to place a cannula and deliver oxygen, which would buy time until a definitive

airway could be created by the insertion of a tracheostomy tube. Sam tilted Mikey's head back further and then
palpated to find the landmark she needed. She swabbed
the area with antiseptic and then reached for a cannula.
Mikey was deeply unconscious now so there was no need
nor time for a local anaesthetic.

Lou was staring with horror at the kit Jake was unrolling on the top of the trolley. The scalpel amongst the
tubes was glinting in the bright light.

'Oh, my God,' she gasped. 'You're not going to cut his
neck, are you? I can't watch.' Her knees were buckling.

The nurse caught her arm. 'Come with me,' she said.
'You don't have to watch.'

Adam moved to follow them but Sam shook her head.
'Stay,' she said. 'Another set of hands would be good.'

Another nurse was sent to upgrade the urgency on the
helicopter backup and it was good to have Adam there as
the controlled chaos of a time-critical invasive procedure
played itself out. Sam inserted the cannula into the neck,
confirmed placement in the trachea and connected the in-
sufflation device. Jake took over delivering the pressured
oxygen in short bursts, monitoring the chest movements
of inhalation and exhalation and drawing up and administering the drugs needed.

Adam watched the monitor, reporting on a rise in oxygen saturation, as he pulled on a pair of gloves and then
used the suction tube and handed Sam what she needed
to make an incision and place a tube instead of the small
cannula to create a stable airway. They were adjusting
the settings on the ventilator when they heard the helicopter coming in to land.

Angus was the lead paramedic on the crew and he

clearly recognised that the tension hadn't dropped much for Sam. Maybe he heard it in her voice as she was giving them the handover of what had been a critical intervention on a paediatric patient who wasn't out of the woods yet.

'Want to come with us,' he asked, 'and keep the continuity of care going? We've got room for both you and mum.'

Jake had brought Lou back into the room.

Sam very much wanted to stay with Mikey until he was safely in the paediatric ICU of a big hospital but...

'Go,' Jake said. 'You've almost finished your shift.'

'But how would I get back?'

'I could follow by road and give you a ride back.'

Adam's quiet voice took Sam by surprise, but when she caught his gaze she realised that not only was he aware of how scary the situation had been for her, he was as deeply invested in the outcome of this case as she was. Mikey was his daughter's best friend. He was the family's GP.

He was part of this.

Sam felt some of the weight of that tension beginning to lift. If there were any warning signs trying to flash that maybe it wasn't a good idea to be alone in a car with Adam Carter for a good hour or more, they were easily ignored.

'Thanks,' Sam said, holding Adam's gaze. 'If it's not a problem for you, that would be really great.'

Adam used some of the road trip to Hamilton to make hands-free phone calls. He'd made a quick call to his mother before he left Coromandel Hospital to make sure she was happy to stay with Charlotte and he'd been to see Janet, who was getting a cast put on her arm, but he needed to talk to her daughter, Claire.

And *his* daughter.

'Why aren't you coming home for dinner, Daddy?'

'Because somebody got really sick and needed to be taken to a big hospital,' he explained.

Adam didn't want to scare Charlotte by telling her that it was Mikey who was sick before he could, hopefully, offer reassurances that her best friend was going to be okay. And if he wasn't, he definitely needed to have that conversation face-to-face with his little girl. Holding her in his arms.

He had to collect himself before saying anything else. 'Dr Sam wanted to go as well, to help take care of them, and they went in the helicopter so I'm going to bring her back home again in the car.'

'Oh…' The sound was one of approval. Clearly, having Dr Sam stuck in another city was enough to create anxiety. 'And then will you come home?'

'Of course I will.'

Adam found himself frowning after he'd ended the call.

Where had *that* come from? Why would Charlie think that being with Sam might mean he wouldn't be coming straight home?

Because he might want to add a detour? To Sam's apartment?

That wasn't going to happen, he reminded himself. Because neither of them wanted it to happen. What was irresistible, however, was the prospect of Sam's company for an hour or more. A chance to talk.

To be in her company.

To get another boost to this new spark that felt like a fuse had been lit in his comfortable—and comforting—

life. A spark that was making him feel more alive than he had in a very long time.

Maybe in forever.

He could hear an echo of Janet Morrison's voice in the back of his head.

'You so deserve to find happiness again after your troubles...and how wonderful would it be for dear little Charlotte to have a mother?'

That wouldn't be Samantha Gillespie, of course, because she'd made it very clear that she didn't do relationships. Or kids. Just like she'd never do a boring job like being a GP again. She'd found the career she wanted to be in for the rest of her life—pre-hospital and retrieval medicine—and nothing was going to stop her achieving that. A relationship could be a barrier to that. Children most certainly would be.

But good on her, Adam thought. How much happier would people be if they were lucky enough to discover what they wanted to do and be and had the means to make it happen?

What they had between them was no more than physical attraction, but maybe it was enough to be the catalyst he'd needed for change in his life? To show *him* that there was something more he might want? Something that would add a whole new dimension to his life that he hadn't realised he was missing so much?

What if this spark that he'd found with Sam could lead to him being open to the possibility of another relationship? That he could, in the not-too-distant future, be a husband as well as a father? That Charlotte could end up having siblings, even?

This was the first time he had considered this to *be* a possibility in the last five years.

This was…huge.

No wonder he could sense emotional red flags that were waving furiously. Or that a part of him was suggesting it would be easier—and safer—to go back to not thinking about it. To stamp on that spark and put it out before it could start a fire and burn something.

But another part was wondering if this might be something too important to destroy.

He did need to think about it, Adam decided. And the only way to be sure he was doing the right thing might be to keep that spark alive for as long as it took to make a decision.

If so, there was no better way to do that than to spend more time in Sam's company.

CHAPTER EIGHT

He was waiting for her outside the hospital.

Leaning against the side of his big SUV, his arms folded.

Smiling at her…

And Sam felt a melting sensation deep inside her body that she'd never felt before.

'Taxi for Dr Gillespie?'

'That would be me.' Sam was smiling back. She walked right up to Adam, stood on tiptoes and kissed him lightly on the lips. 'Thank you so much for doing this.'

'It's my pleasure.' Adam opened the passenger door for her. 'How's Mikey doing?'

'Stable. Sedated and ventilated. He's had a chest X-ray to confirm correct placement of the tracheostomy tube. He's on broad-spectrum antibiotics and steroids to reduce swelling for the next twenty-four to forty-eight hours.' Sam pulled her safety belt over her shoulder. 'His mum and dad are beside his bed and he'll be monitored continuously in ICU. He's as safe as he can be.'

Adam got behind the wheel and started the car. 'That was one of the most adrenaline-loaded situations I've ever been a part of. Even more so than that accident scene was.' His sideways glance at Sam was one of admiration. 'Exciting, but I don't think I'd want to chase it as a career. Or do it every day, even. It would be exhausting. Are you tired now?'

'No.' Sam threw him a grin. 'I'm a bit wired, to be honest. And hungry. *Really* hungry. Could we possibly stop at a fast-food restaurant and get some horribly unhealthy burgers?'

Adam laughed. 'Sure. I know one that's on the outskirts of town. Not that I'm admitting to possibly having been there before or anything.'

He focused on his driving for the next few minutes to get through the heavy big-city traffic of people heading home. Sam found herself watching his profile and thinking about…adrenaline.

She was still buzzing from the emergency and the helicopter journey and being involved in the rapid decision-making and actions in the intensive care unit. What was standing out to her right now, however, was the moment it had begun. When Mikey had stopped breathing and Adam had caught her gaze for a heartbeat before jumping off the edge of the bed to help her begin the resuscitation.

She'd felt that connection before, when they'd been working together at that major accident scene and treating Jason.

And when she'd come out of the main doors of this city hospital to find him waiting for her, she'd known what it was that made their rapport different. Adam had her back. He was caring for *her* at the same time he was caring for their patient. It was dangerous territory because it was breaking boundaries of being colleagues or friends, even.

This was the kind of space where people could fall properly in love and that was…

Unthinkable, that was what it was.

If it happened, it could derail everything Sam had been working towards for years. She only needed to remind herself of that to be quite confident she would never let it happen—any more than she would allow herself to get pregnant and welcome a baby into the world. If anything, today had reminded her of how much in love with her job she was and that nothing could compete with that.

But she was still full of adrenaline.

And *so* hungry…

Double meat, double cheese, extra sauce and jalapeños. Large fries. The token salad in the bun did nothing to stop this being a disgustingly unhealthy meal.

But Adam had to admit it tasted pretty good.

Even better, was watching Sam wolf her food down with such enjoyment. They hadn't gone into the overly bright, crowded restaurant. He'd taken them through the drive-through and Sam held the fragrant paper bags on her lap until he'd driven far enough to get to a picnic area just out of the city, off the motorway. They sat in the car and ate. As Sam finished her burger, she licked some melted cheese off her fingers and Adam could feel every cell in his body responding.

This woman was *so* damn sexy…

He needed to move. To distract himself so that he would be able to focus on the road when they got going again. He got out of the car to take their rubbish to a bin that was provided near a picnic table. He didn't realise that Sam had followed him until he turned and there she was, right in front of him—a smile playing with the corners of her mouth and her eyes shining. She looked as though she was still as wired as she had been when he'd picked her up. Looking for a bit more excitement, perhaps?

Yes…he saw the way the tip of her tongue appeared and moistened her lips. 'Are you a fan of outdoor sex?' she asked softly.

'I wouldn't know,' Adam had to confess 'I've never tried it.'

Sam's eyes widened. 'Really? What about back seat of car sex?'

'Nope.' Adam was feeling slightly embarrassed now. He suspected that Sam had experienced it all in her exciting world.

Her voice was even quieter now. 'How lucky are you?'

'What do you mean?'

'The first time is quite possibly the best. Definitely the time you'll never forget.'

Oh…dear Lord… Adam had a feeling he didn't need to answer the question about how lucky he was. Instead, he asked one himself, his voice a raw growl.

'Your choice… Back seat or the bushes?'

Sam looked thoughtful. Then she reached out with her hand and when Adam took hold of it, she pulled him into the greenery, well out of sight of any of the traffic rushing past on the motorway.

Moments later, Adam was holding Sam's face between his hands, kissing her senseless as she leaned back against a tree. He couldn't even hear the traffic now because he was being pulled into the fastest, *hottest* sex he'd ever had. Kisses that felt almost desperate. The touch of skin on skin with the brush of leaves and shifting clothing putting every sense onto a new level. The heat of desire, the taste of Sam's mouth and the feel of her breast in his hand. The sounds of need—and exquisite pleasure—that they both uttered. The scent of sex that made it impossible to think clearly. It was over in minutes but they were both breathless. And smiling…

'That was fun,' Sam said.

Fun? It had been mind-blowing as far as Adam was concerned but he gave a huff of laughter that sounded like agreement.

'Sorry.' Sam's expression was contrite. 'That wasn't supposed to happen again, was it?'

'I'm not complaining,' Adam said.

'Hmm…' She was frowning now. 'It's all good fun until someone loses an eye, isn't it?' Her glance held a warning. 'This doesn't change anything, okay? This can't get serious, Adam.'

'It won't.' The promise was heartfelt. He wasn't about to risk his heart, let alone Charlotte's.

But it felt non-negotiable that this wasn't going to happen again. It wasn't even occurring to him to suggest the possibility.

Because it had been more than mere fun?

Because he was getting a taste of what it was like to be as wild as Sam was?

Because he liked feeling like this?

Being in Sam's orbit was a completely different planet. Adrenaline-filled medical scenarios and the kind of sex he'd only seen in the movies or read about in a steamy novel.

Wild.

Thank goodness it was only temporary, Adam thought as they walked back to the car. He doubted that he could keep up this kind of pace in either his professional or personal life but there was no way he wasn't going to make the most of it while he could. He just needed to think of a way to see more of Sam while still keeping it private and avoiding any long-lasting complications.

'I'm thinking of joining LandSAR as a volunteer.'

Sam blinked. 'Really?'

'Yes. It's good if they have a doctor as part of a team, isn't it?'

Sam nodded. 'Absolutely.'

'And you're not going to be here forever, are you?'

Sam shook her head this time. 'No helicopter crews to join around here. I'll be hunting for a job in a major centre. Auckland, Wellington, Christchurch. Maybe Australia.' She could hear the excitement in her own voice. Her dream career was getting closer every day. With the prospect of completing her training visibly on the horizon now, she could start looking for, and perhaps even applying for, any positions that were advertised.

'So they might be happy to have me join the team,' Adam suggested. 'I might not be available that often, but I'd be happy to be on call.'

'I'm sure Colin would be delighted to have you,' Sam said. But then she frowned. 'You'd have to give up a few evenings or even a weekend here and there to do some training, though. That's time away from Charlie.'

'More time with her gran. They'd both be happy with that. I think Mum would be even happier that I was doing something for the community as well. And for myself?' Adam was smiling at her. 'It's always good to learn something new. What sort of training would I be doing?'

Sam blew out a breath. 'There's a foundation course to

get through first. Navigation skills, using maps and GPS. Communication stuff with radios and tracking software. Search methods, survival skills, ropes...' She was counting the categories off on her fingers. 'There are lectures, practical sessions, real scenarios in all sorts of different terrains. It would take a month or two before you were up to speed to officially join a real search.'

Adam nodded. 'So when could I start?'

'I'll talk to Colin. He's a fire officer so we get to use the training room facilities at the station. He'll probably give you some reading to do on the structure and roles within search and rescue. With a bit of luck there'll be a fresh intake for volunteers starting soon and it's about time I got involved in more than teaching only the first aid sessions.'

Things fell into place with a speed that suggested they were meant to be, and it was after the first evening of a new foundation course at the fire station that Sam realised just how inspired Adam's decision to sign up for joining the organisation had been. This was a totally legitimate reason for them to be spending time together and the fire station was on her side of town. It was only polite for Adam to offer her a lift home and that gave them the kind of time together that neither of them seemed to be able to get enough of.

One week led to another and another. Colin was delighted with the proficiency that Adam was showing in every aspect of his training.

'We'll get Doc Carter sorted with a uniform,' he told Sam. 'With the head start he already had with his tramping experience and medical skills, he could be deployed for any daytime searches from now on, I think. Oh, and Sam?'

'Yes?'

'There's a school fair coming up which is always a big community event so we like to have a presence and usually have a stand to show off some of our gear and keep up our visibility for future fundraising. Can we count on you to help out for an hour or two on the day?'

'Sure. Just let me know the date. As long as I'm not on duty, I'll be there.'

Sam's first experience of talking to that large group of young children at the local primary school, in the wake of some of them being rescued from their forest outing, had turned out to be much more fun than she had expected. A memorable day all round, in fact, ending up with her having dinner at Adam's house and that first kiss.

Oh yeah... Sam was never going to forget that kiss. Or anything else that had happened between them since then. It gave her a delicious tingle just thinking about it and that only added to the delights of her first traditional school fair that was an extraordinary mix of shopping, activities and pure fun. No wonder the huge crowd of people looked so happy and the vibe was inclusive and so upbeat.

The time she'd spent with Colin in front of the LandSAR posters showing dramatic rescue scenes, with their stretchers, packs and other gear around them, talking to parents and children about the work they did, had flown past. A surprising number of people, both children and adults, had recognised her. It wasn't only the children and their parents who'd met her at school that day that wanted to stop and chat. There were people who'd met her in the emergency department of the hospital, as patients or relatives.

'You looked after my dad, Jonno Peters, when he had

a heart attack,' a middle-aged woman said. 'Do you remember?'

'Yes, I do. We sent him off in a helicopter, didn't we? I heard he did very well.'

'He's still doing great. He says he's had a rebore with those stents and there's no stopping him now.'

'I'll never forget how kind you were,' someone else told her. 'I was so scared that I was going to die. That pain was worse than childbirth.'

'Renal colic is probably number one of the worst pains you can get,' Sam agreed. 'I'm not surprised you were scared.'

'You made me feel so much better. Thank you.'

'You're so welcome.'

Mikey's mother was here, but couldn't stop to talk. 'I'm manning the cake stall,' she told Sam. She held up a tin. 'And I've made a couple of my famous chocolate mud cakes. Want me to put one aside for you?'

'Ooh, yes, please. How's Mikey?'

'Lining up for a pony ride. He's with his nana.'

The little boy who could have died that day from epiglottitis had bounced back after his stay in ICU. That had been a great day, too, Sam thought as she watched Mikey's mum hurry away. Not just for the dramatic medical emergency that had turned out so well, but for Adam's part in the day and that brief but very memorable stop on the way home.

'It's Dr *Sam*!' Children pointed at her and Sam waved back. How cool was it that she knew so many people even though she hadn't worked here for very long? And that they made her feel appreciated. Part of the community, even.

Charlie, wearing her Supergirl outfit over jeans and sneakers, ran up for a hug when she came past with Adam, closely followed by Jake and Isla, who were with someone Sam hadn't seen for months.

'*Arlo*. When did you get so tall?'

The boy grinned but ducked his head, reaching down to pat the dog by his side as if Ben the border collie was his touchstone.

'Can you come with us, Sam?' Charlie begged. 'We're going to ride the ponies.'

Adam was introducing Colin to Jake and Isla but he turned and smiled at Sam.

'You go,' he told her. 'I can hold the fort here. You probably haven't been to a school fair like this before. Go and enjoy.'

Charlotte was beside Arlo now, looking up at the older boy with what looked like hero worship. Arlo was Jake's nephew. And the nephew that Isla hadn't known *she* had. Sam had watched her colleagues from a distance last year, as they'd navigated not only their unexpected roles as parents to Arlo but their growing feelings for each other. They were a tight family unit now, even though it had, apparently, been the last thing either of them had seen in their futures. Sam couldn't imagine it.

Or could she?

It was too easy to be in the moment and enjoy this company and everything happening around them.

Happy groups of people were perusing stalls where there were plants for sale alongside homemade crafts and baking. Adam's mother, Jude, was in charge of selling beautifully bottled jars of jam and chutney. Raffle tickets were being sold and children were eagerly waiting their turn for face painting, temporary tattoos or hair braid-ing. Sam could see a bouncy castle in the distance and a tractor providing rides as an alternative to the line-up of patient shaggy ponies being led around in circles.

Jake and Isla paused to look at the white elephant stall with tables covered with a vast array of second-hand items for sale. Jake picked up a small ball and Ben's attention was instantly caught. Isla laughed.

'Ball is life,' she said. 'And we so need another ball in the garden.'

'I'll buy it,' Arlo said. 'I've got my pocket money.'

'Can I throw it for Ben?' Charlotte asked.

'Okay… I'll show you what to do.' Arlo led them away from the stalls and Sam could see him making sure Ben waited patiently for the ball to be thrown.

Jake had spotted a sausage sizzle beside other food carts. 'I'm *starving*,' he told Isla. 'Is it time for lunch?'

'Absolutely. Let's join the queue.' Isla looked over her shoulder. 'Sam? Want a sausage? Or hot chips?'

'Ooh…hot chips sound great. Thank you. We'll watch the kids.'

'We'll get some food for them, too. We can have a picnic.'

Sam stayed beside Adam as she watched her colleagues move to the queue. Someone walked past them balancing a sausage wrapped in bread and smothered with tomato sauce in one hand and a pottle of hot chips in the other and Sam found her gaze locked on the chips. Would she ever see this ubiquitous item of food without remember-ing that first night with Adam?

Sitting on her bed, eating fish and chips after the best sex of her life. Talking to the man who'd stolen a piece of her heart that night by simply holding her in his arms.

Her thoughts were broken by the tug on her hand. 'Did you see, Sam? Did you see how far I could throw the ball for Ben?'

Oh… Charlotte was looking up at her with the same kind of look she had been giving Arlo a few minutes ago. A look that suggested the answer to her question might be the most important thing in the world right now.

'I'm sorry, sweetheart, I didn't see,' Sam apologised. 'Show me again?'

Charlotte grinned and ran back to Arlo and Ben. Both Sam and Adam watched her pick up the ball and laughed at the way Ben backed away slowly, his eyes on the prize, ready to run or catch the ball at any moment.

Sam had the strangest feeling that she was looking down at this scene. A man and woman standing watching children play—like so many other families here today. And she could move further away and see the whole community coming together to support a school's fundraising event and…and she was part of it. It felt like home.

It felt like family.

But it also felt like the anchor that was the last thing she wanted in her life and Sam could feel an edge of panic hovering.

'Watch!' Charlotte shouted.

'We're watching,' Adam called back.

Charlotte put all her effort into throwing the ball but it didn't go very far at all. Ben didn't seem to mind. He leapt to catch it and then took it back to lay it carefully beside the foot of a little girl who was bursting with pride as she looked back at them.

Sam could feel Adam's gaze on her and turned her head to find an odd expression on his face.

Could he sense the deep unease she was feeling?

Was he feeling it himself?

'Charlie adores you,' he said quietly. 'I can only imagine how much worse it's going to be when you leave if she gets any idea of what's going on between us.'

Sam could see the way the muscles in his throat moved as he swallowed. 'This wasn't supposed to happen,' he added, almost to himself.

And here it was. The chance to disrupt that disconcerting idea that she was in a place that felt like home. With people who were starting to feel far too much like family. That she might be responsible for making a little girl unhappy.

A little girl that it would be far too easy to start loving too much.

She chose her words carefully, as if she was testing how they would sound. Maybe Sam was hoping that sharing the words might somehow make it easier. They'd both known this was going to happen eventually, after all. She was just making the call because she'd heard the sound of an alarm that couldn't be ignored.

'Maybe it's time to stop,' she said quietly.

There was a long, long moment of silence as they watched Arlo throw the ball for Ben, Charlotte clapping with glee as the dog ran to catch it, his excited bark a joyous sound.

And then Adam spoke, his gaze not shifting from his daughter.

'Yeah…' His voice sounded rough. 'I hate the idea, but I think that's exactly what we have to do.'

CHAPTER NINE

IT MIGHT HAVE been easier to get past missing the private time he'd had with Sam if he wasn't spending any time at all with her, but he couldn't allow himself to give in to the last-minute temptation, no matter how powerful it was, of finding an excuse not to go to the LandSAR training session a few days after the school fair.

Adam Carter had never been the kind of person to commit to something and then simply walk away from it and he wasn't about to start now.

Being indecisive had led to him being almost late, however. When he arrived at the fire station, the other local volunteers who were going through the foundation course were already seated. Colin Smythe was at the foot of the long table, connecting his laptop to the large screen on the wall. He looked up and smiled broadly when he saw Adam enter the room.

'Take a seat,' he invited. 'I'm about to show you all what a game-changer it is to have tracking software available.'

But Adam hesitated. There was only one empty chair left at the table. 'Shall I find another chair?'

'Nah…you're the last one we were waiting for.' Colin's sideways glance made Adam realise that his thoughts had been transparent. 'Sam can't make it this evening,' he said. 'I believe she's got an online interview for a job that might be coming up in Wellington. Or was it Auckland?' He tapped the mouse pad on his laptop and a complicated-looking map with gridlines and dots and all sorts of sidebars and inserts filled the screen. Colin was smiling as he looked up again. 'It's great timing that you've decided to join us, Adam. We'd be fretting about losing our top medic on the crew otherwise.'

Adam sat down in the empty space at the table, responding to greetings from the others on autopilot.

Sam was applying for a new job?

She was *leaving*?

Was it because she had also been tempted by the idea that it would be easier to put an end to their albeit undefined relationship by simply avoiding *his* company?

That didn't quite make sense. Sam was the one who'd suggested it was time that they stopped seeing each other. She'd been the one who'd reminded him that it could never be anything serious, so it was hard to imagine that she was finding going back to the life she'd had before she'd met him was messing with her head space the way it was with his. He'd been so sure that this was only *his* problem.

'Back in the day,' Colin told them all, 'we'd be running a search with a whiteboard in the ops tent, marker pens and an eraser and half a dozen radios that were scattered all over the place, out in the bush. This app isn't just a GPS tracker, it lets us see where everyone is, in real time. What we've covered, what we haven't and whether any clues have been found.'

Adam tried to focus, but it wasn't easy.

He was still thinking about Sam. He couldn't stop thinking about her, to be honest, even though he knew he had to protect his daughter from getting too close to someone who was always going to leave a place and a job that wasn't exciting enough for her.

He understood why she had to leave.

Sam had brought a whole new spark into his life. While for him it was enough to merely experience the glow from the edges, he could understand the pull of the adrenaline rush of rescue work and critically ill patients instead of the standard fare of far more mundane family medicine cases. He was envious of Sam's ability to keep boundaries in her personal life so that she wouldn't have obstacles to being the person she wanted to be.

But was he right in wondering whether her absence this evening was partly due to finding it easier to avoid him? And that looking for a new job was, perhaps, a more definitive way to cope? Was it ever that simple for anyone to have the kind of intimate relationship they'd been having without it becoming significant? And, if so…was there a chance that a different outcome wasn't beyond the realms of possibility?

Adam tried to push away something that was undoubtedly no more than wishful thinking. He focused on what Colin was saying.

'You can see that everything is recorded and time stamped. All radio traffic and updates. This is crucial because if the job ends up with a fatality, it could be months before the Coroner's Court look into the case and make potential recommendations for what could be done to prevent future disasters. You won't remember why you made a call to change something at four a.m. in the pouring rain but it'll all be recorded here.' He looked around the group. 'That time stamping can help keep *you* safe as well. If you get injured and stop moving, we'll be able to get to you faster.'

Some of his words echoed in Adam's head.

Keeping safe…

That was what he had been trying to do right from the start, when that overwhelming attraction to Samantha Gillespie had come out of nowhere and threatened to derail the life he'd built over the last five years.

He'd been trying to keep Charlotte safe.

And that meant he was also keeping himself safe.

He knew he would be doing the right thing by letting Sam go, and that included any fantasies about how they might, somehow, be able to make it work so that this new hole in his life could be repaired.

It just didn't *feel* like the right thing.

She only had herself to blame.

Sam reminded herself of this fact every time she felt the pang of missing Adam Carter. When she could hear echoes of his voice or his laughter and imagine that steady gaze catching hers and, maybe the hardest of all, imagined his touch as she lay alone in her bed every night.

It was her own fault that she'd let it happen in the first place, of course, although she couldn't blame herself for that. Who wouldn't have given in to an attraction that was so powerful it would have been a struggle *not* to allow yourself to give in to its magnetic pull, at least once? It was only supposed to have been a kiss. Just to see if there had really been something so very different about this man.

And, dammit, there *had* been.

Something different enough to make her wonder what it would be like to have the opportunity to step a little closer. To do more than simply experience the most amazing kiss ever.

That difference had been enough for her to have invited him to come to her house that night to eat his fish and chip dinner.

And that was supposed to have been the end of it. Just one night. Nothing that was going to damage the boundaries in their lives that they were both determined to protect for very good reasons.

What was it about fast food? Hamburgers had played their part in what could only be seen as the biggest mistake she'd made. That tacit agreement that they could keep seeing each other because they'd both promised that it would never become anything serious.

It still *wasn't* serious. Adam wasn't going to let anyone close enough to his daughter to risk damaging her life and Sam wasn't about to give up her dream career and step into a role as a wife and—the thought sent a chill down her spine—a *mother*?

So why did it feel serious? Why did her thoughts keep circling back to Adam Carter? Was it really her own fault that she was struggling with this distraction?

Yeah…she only had herself to blame for how she was feeling now, but it was only a couple of weeks after the school fair and she was at least doing something about fixing things. She had taken the first definitive step towards getting herself out of a predicament she really didn't want to be in, when she'd used her network last week to ask about any upcoming jobs at the major helicopter rescue services both in New Zealand and Australia. This week, things were starting to move a lot faster than she had expected. They'd taken on a momentum that would be difficult to stop, in fact. Pretty soon, it would be a done deal and her time with Adam would only be a memory. And that was a good thing, wasn't it?

Sam was still considering the repercussions of a decision she'd made only yesterday evening when she was walking to one of the computers in the central hub of Coromandel Hospital's emergency department. She went past Jess, the nurse on triage duty, who was picking up a phone that provided a direct link for ambulance crews to use.

'Receiving you loud and clear,' she heard Jess say. 'Go ahead...' She listened for a moment, scribbling a note on a piece of paper. 'Roger that,' she said. Then, 'What's your ETA?'

Sam had given up on her plan to chase down some lab results. 'What's coming in?' she asked Jess.

'Status two patient,' Jess said. 'Ninety-five-year-old woman with a ruptured varicose vein in her calf. Significant blood loss. Estimated Stage Two hypovolaemic shock—tachycardic and hypotensive. Bleeding's still not under control. GCS fourteen.'

'Right...' Sam was thinking fast. 'We're going to need warmed IV fluids and blankets in Resus. What's the ETA?'

'Three minutes.'

'Okay. Call the blood bank, would you please, Jess, and put them on standby for activating a major haemorrhage protocol. Where's Jake?'

'Still in CT with the girl who crashed her bike.'

Sam nodded. She'd helped with the resuscitation of the bike rider who'd been clipped by a truck on the main road so she knew the young woman might have a critical head injury. She would need to handle this case without the other emergency department consultant on duty. 'Call in anyone else on the trauma team who's available, please. I'm going to need some help.'

Assistance from another doctor *was* available as her patient arrived but it came from the last person Sam might have expected. Striding beside the stretcher, his hands keeping pressure on a wad of dressing on the elderly woman's lower leg that was elevated on pillows, was Adam Carter.

For just a split second Sam was overwhelmed by the rush of emotion that came from seeing him for the first time since the day of the school fair. It was far more than the relief of knowing she had competent professional assistance available. This feeling was a very personal relief. Elation, almost, that she could feel rushing through her veins like the most powerful IV drug ever discovered. Something so personal that Sam knew she had to push it aside instantly. Effectively enough to make it disappear completely. She couldn't allow anything—or any*one*—to interfere with the focus she needed for her patient right now.

'This is Janet Morrison,' the paramedic relayed. 'She had a fall in her garden approximately twenty minutes ago and got a puncture wound in her leg from a sharp stick that has ruptured a large varicose vein. Her daughter was in the house. She put pressure on the wound with a towel and called her doctor for advice. The medical centre's just down the road so Dr Carter got there within a couple of minutes.'

'Hi, Janet.' Sam picked up one of Janet's hands, noting how cold and clammy it was. 'I'm Sam, one of the doctors here. Do you remember me? I was on duty when Dr Carter brought you in not so long ago after you broke your wrist.'

Janet's voice was muffled by the mask but she nodded. She still looked frightened, however. And confused, which was probably why her level of consciousness had been a point down from normal.

Sam gave her hand a reassuring squeeze and smiled at her. 'We're going to take really good care of you,' she promised.

'I'm Claire.' A grey-haired woman was holding Janet's other hand. 'I'm her daughter. Can I stay with her?'

'Of course you can.' She looked up at the ambulance crew. 'Let's get her onto our bed. On my count?' She caught Adam's gaze. 'Can you keep the pressure on while we move her?' At his nod, she started counting. 'One, two...three...'

It felt as if their patient weighed almost nothing. A warming mattress was already on the bed and there were blankets from the warmer waiting to cover her. The nurses and ambulance crew worked to change the monitoring equipment from portable to departmental. The blood pressure cuff, oxygen saturation monitor and electrodes relaying information about Janet's heart rate and rhythm were quickly swapped. The tubing providing oxygen to her mask was plugged into one of the overhead inlets.

Sam watched the numbers appearing on the monitor screen. Janet's heart rate was too fast and her blood pressure too low. She was pale and her breathing was rapid and shallow.

'We weren't able to get IV access,' the paramedic apologised. 'She's shut down and Dr Carter thought it was better to get here as fast as possible. We estimated the initial blood loss to be about a litre.'

Sam nodded. 'Good call.'

She gave a few rapid instructions to the nursing staff to gather everything she needed to get a line in. They would need to warm Janet up for a short time and then she would use ultrasound guidance and have one attempt at a peripheral line. If that failed, she'd need to go for an intraosseous line or a central venous one if there was enough time. It was urgent to be able to administer drugs and infuse fluids and blood products to counteract the shock that could easily be fatal.

'Any past history I should know about?' she asked.

'Hypertension, high cholesterol, angina and Type Two diabetes,' Adam responded.

'On any blood thinners?'

'No.'

She looked at the pressure Adam was still putting on the dressing over the wound. 'Are you okay to keep the pressure on until we've got IV access for fluids and some tranexamic acid on board?'

His nod told her that he understood the danger of Janet losing any more blood. His pressure might be stopping the flow but, even without being on blood thinners, the mechanisms for clotting to be effective could be reduced in dilated varicose veins, with valves that weren't functioning well and low blood pressure already reducing circulation.

The eye contact he made with her at the same time gave her another one of those tiny moments of lost focus as Sam reached for a pair of sterile gloves and pulled them on. No more than a flash of time that no one else would have been aware of, but it was long enough for a whole kaleidoscope of thoughts and feelings to coalesce in her brain and body before they were dismissed.

It had only taken a glance.

Because that connection was *so* strong. It didn't seem to matter what had led to the direct eye contact—attraction, empathy, a professional exchange or simply pleasure in them being in the same space—the effect was undeniable. A way of communicating that was as rare as it was dangerous.

She should have run for the hills the first time she'd felt it, when she'd told Adam how sorry she was for him losing his wife so tragically and he'd looked straight into her soul and seen that she knew what that kind of grief was like, way before she'd told him anything about Robbie.

But how seductive had it been, on a whole other level than anything physical, to feel as if someone could really *see* you?

And that you mattered?

Yes. This was her own fault that she was standing here on the edge of a cliff and she could see that dark chasm below her that was the place you fell into when you lost the person that mattered the most to you.

Someone you loved. The way she knew it would be possible to love Adam Carter. And Charlotte.

Sam couldn't do that again.

She wouldn't let herself do that again.

Adam was staring at Sam's back as she pulled on a pair of gloves and arranged what she needed around her to try and get an IV line into Janet Morrison. He could sense the tension in her body as if he was feeling it himself and the urge to touch her in comfort or reassurance was strong enough to make him blink. He couldn't move, of course, and he wouldn't have done anything more than offer support with a glance, but the power of that urge was disturbing.

If he'd needed any proof that distance was needed between himself and Sam, this was it.

That need to touch her was filling his heart. He could even feel it in his fingertips and it was powerful enough to be taking his breath away.

There was only one reason that he was feeling like this.

He loved Sam.

He was *in* love with her.

He wanted to share her joy, comfort her sadness and smooth away her stress. He wanted her to know that he would always have her back. That he would be there, no matter what. For as long as he had breath in his body. Because he loved her.

And he couldn't let her know any of that.

Because she didn't want that in her life. He couldn't try and change her mind either, because how much of a risk would that be? How could he even think of persuading someone to stay when the risk that the choice had been made under pressure—and wasn't what she *really* wanted—would always be there? Hanging over him but, more importantly, hanging over Charlotte.

He couldn't do it.

He *wouldn't* do it.

By the time she turned around, that impression that she was less than confident was completely gone. And any urge to give her even a reassuring glance had also evaporated.

He watched the skill with which she held the ultrasound transducer in her left hand, the white walls of the veins clearly visible on the screen, and the needle of the cannula in her right hand. Adam could see the care she took in advancing the needle into the centre of the vein. He could even see the tiny plastic catheter being pushed gently into place before the ultrasound transducer was discarded, no longer needed. With the plug securing the end of the line, a blood sample was taken and rushed off for a type and cross-match, drugs to help combat blood loss were given and warm fluids were hung to start replacing lost volume.

The skill and swiftness with which Sam had accomplished what could have been a difficult challenge was no surprise. Neither was the rest of her care of his patient. Adam's role in the management of his patient was no longer needed as he finally released the pressure he'd been keeping on the wound and they found the bleeding was under control, but when he tried to leave, Janet became distressed.

'Please don't go, Dr Carter,' the old woman pleaded. '*You're* my doctor…'

That note of certainty in Janet's voice brought back, once again, the memory of something else she'd said to him.

'You so deserve to find happiness again after your troubles…and how wonderful would it be for dear little Charlotte to have a mother?'

That had been what had persuaded him to spend more time with Sam when he knew perfectly well it wasn't the best idea. But he recognised the new spark that had entered his life and it had felt like more than simply his body coming alive again. It had felt like…hope—that one day he could be open to another relationship because Sam was showing him how much joy it could add to his life? And how much it could add to Charlotte's life to have a mother because that big heart in her little body made it so easy for her to love the women who were important to her. Her gamma. Miss Kempsey. Dr Sam the superhero…

Right from the start he'd known it couldn't be Sam.

But now he knew it couldn't be anyone *other* than Sam.

Because he was in love with her. Because the spark that she had brought into his life couldn't possibly be transferred to anyone else because it didn't exist on its own.

Samantha Gillespie had created it. She *was* that spark. And when she walked out of his life she would be taking it with her.

He couldn't pretend that the way she was smiling at him in this moment was any encouragement. This was purely professional. Her next words proved that.

'You are Janet's primary doctor,' she said. 'Please stay, if you can.'

So he did. Because stress could make Janet's condition worse and possibly even contribute to renewed bleeding before the damage to the vein could be repaired. Blood products arrived and were infused, and Janet's vital signs began to show significant improvement. By the time the surgeon arrived in the emergency department to see Janet before she was taken to Theatre, both Janet and Claire were clearly feeling a great deal happier.

But Adam wasn't.

He was still there when Janet was wheeled away to Theatre and her daughter was taken to a relatives' room to wait. Nurses were busy tidying the resuscitation room, moving in and out with equipment and supplies that needed cleaning or replacing, and he waited for a moment alone with Sam to excuse himself and get back to his medical centre. He needed to escape. To try and clear his head from what had been both revealing and more than a little devastating.

'Good job,' he told her. 'Janet was lucky that you were on duty this morning.'

Sam smiled at him. 'She's lucky to have you for her GP and that you got to her so fast. The outcome could have been very different.'

Her gaze seemed to slide away from his as she spoke and Adam felt a tiny chill tickle his spine.

'You okay?' he asked quietly.

'I'm good.' Sam's tone was bright. 'I got offered a job last night—as a HEMS doctor on a helicopter crew based in Wellington.'

'Wow…' Adam's smile felt forced. 'Your dream job.'

This was it. The end was rushing towards him. Even if he had the courage to take that risk of bringing someone else into his—and Charlotte's—life, he also knew that it was something that Sam would never even want to consider.

He couldn't tell her how he felt. The only thing that would achieve would be to take some of the shine of the glow of the future that was waiting for her elsewhere. The job that she'd been working towards for so long.

Sam was smiling back at him. 'It's only a locum position for now, but it could become permanent if I'm a good fit.'

'How could you not be?' Adam's smile was poignant now. 'What did you tell them?'

Sam wasn't meeting his gaze. 'I said yes,' she said softly. She cleared her throat and looked up. 'Like you said, it's my dream job. How could I turn it down?'

It had to be his imagination, but Adam could actually feel something shifting beneath him, almost as if a sinkhole was beginning to form.

'How long?' he asked. 'Before you leave?'

CHAPTER TEN

TWO WEEKS.

Fourteen days.

Long enough to thank the friends she'd made amongst her colleagues at Coromandel Hospital and the people in the community she had worked with. She shouted a round of drinks at a local pub after the next Wednesday night training session with the LandSAR team and the new volunteers.

For the first time since he'd started the course, Adam hadn't made it that evening and Sam had been acutely aware of his absence from the moment she'd walked through the door of the training room, carrying a box of splints, bandages and slings. She was going to give the volunteers a crash course in identifying and stabilising potential fractures if they were first on the scene before any medics arrived.

'Did Adam say anything, Colin? About why he wouldn't be here?'

Colin shook his head. 'I don't think it was anything planned. I saw him yesterday to give him the rest of his uniform and gear and he didn't mention it then. I only got the message ten minutes ago to apologise that he couldn't make it tonight.'

If Adam knew what was on the agenda, he might well have decided to give it a miss because he certainly didn't need any first aid training but…he would be taking over this kind of session when she left so why wouldn't he want to take part as a trial run? She couldn't help feeling worried now. Had something happened?

Was Charlotte not well? Or Jude? Was Adam caring for the most important people in his life or were they caring for him? The thought that it might be Adam who was sick gave Sam a squeeze in her chest that made her catch her breath.

'He did say he'd definitely be here again next week,' Colin added.

When she wouldn't be here?

She couldn't blame him if it was deliberate. What was surprising was how sad it would be if he did feel the need to avoid her company. It had been a reluctant but mutual decision to stop seeing each other, but surely that didn't mean they couldn't be friends and keep in touch in the future? The connection they'd discovered wasn't going to disappear and Sam would be delighted to get updates on how Charlotte was doing as she grew up and how happy Adam was with his life. She'd want to know if he'd been on any exciting search and rescue missions and he would be the one she'd want to share her own stories with.

Sam started setting out examples of items that could be used if commercial air, malleable or padded splints weren't available. Short tree branches. A magazine. A cushion and the side of a cardboard box. She had a whole bag of crepe bandages that they'd use later to practise immobilising an arm or ankle.

That sense of missing Adam wasn't going away in a hurry. Neither was her concern, so maybe it was just as well Adam *wasn't* here. The fact that Sam couldn't get this nagging disquiet out of her mind was a very clear alarm bell sounding. She'd allowed her relationship with Adam to not only cross boundaries but to get to a space she'd vowed to never find herself in again.

The space where the happiness and wellbeing of someone else could actually seem more important than your own.

The space where you could only be when you loved someone *that* much.

The discomfort associated with that tight sensation that made it hard to take a breath was similar to having a piece of skin torn off, Sam decided as she straightened a professional splint where layers of dense foam sandwiched a pliable sheet of aluminium.

Or was that pain more like feeling a piece of your heart breaking off?

Whatever. It advertised loss. Not just the kind of loss of leaving friends behind whose company she would miss, like Jake and Isla or countless others in her past that she remembered fondly from all the jobs she'd had and the many places she'd lived. This felt like it wasn't going to turn into a happy memory. It had the potential to be a pocket of grief that would always feel raw.

Because she didn't just care about Adam Carter.

Somehow, she had missed the safety barriers. Allowed herself to be seduced by the impression that it was safe because they were both on the same page and it was only ever going to be temporary.

What Sam had done, she realised, was to fall in love with Adam.

For the first time in her life, she had fallen head over heels in love with someone.

Oh, she still carried the pain of losing Robbie because of how much she'd loved him, but she hadn't been *in* love with him. He'd been her best friend and by far the most important person in her world, and perhaps it would have grown into an adult kind of relationship, but it had never had the chance to become more than a bond between soulmates. She'd never discovered what it might be like to be physically intimate with someone you connected with at that kind of level.

And she'd never let herself connect with anyone else like that again.

Until now.

It felt as if she'd never had the choice, really. That connection had simply been there, right from the moment she'd met Adam, and resistance had proved too easy to excuse.

Adam's avoidance of her since last week when she'd told him she was leaving seemed to suggest that he might be finding this difficult as well but, even if he was prepared to accept the risk of a relationship in his own life, he had made it clear he wasn't prepared to accept that risk on Charlotte's behalf. There was only one thing she could do that might make this easier for both of them. She could work out her notice and then take herself away from this place and its people.

Maybe what they both needed was to move on as soon as possible.

The call came when Adam was making a house call to a patient who'd just returned home after surgery and a stay in hospital.

He had just finished taking Janet Morrison's blood pressure.

'Back to normal,' he said. 'Just like your heart rate and oxygen saturation and everything else I've checked. You're a bit of a legend, Janet, but you're going to need to take it easy for a bit longer. I don't want to see you out in your garden any time soon.'

'No chance of that.' Janet's daughter, Claire, came into the sitting room, where her mother was on the couch, her leg elevated on a cushion and encased in a compression stocking. She put a tray down that had a teapot in a knitted cosy, several cups and saucers and a heaped plate of what looked like homemade shortbread. 'We're just here for a day or two to pack, then we're back to Hamilton. Mum's going to stay with us until she's recuperated properly.'

The glance Adam received told him that there were bigger decisions to be made in the near future about where Janet was going to be living.

'Sounds good,' he said. 'Let me know if I can be of any help, won't you?'

'Thanks.' Claire was setting pretty cups with a pattern of red roses onto matching saucers. 'Have you got time for a cup of tea, Dr Carter?'

It was at that point that his phone beeped with a text message and Claire shook her head. 'I expect that suggests you haven't.'

Adam's eyes widened as he scanned his phone. 'It's my first official LandSAR callout,' he told them. 'An alarm's been raised because a tramper's gone missing on a descent from the Pinnacles Hut.'

'Ooh…there's some rugged country up there,' Janet said.

'There is,' Adam agreed. 'I went up the first time with my dad when I was only eight years old and the metal rungs to get up the cliff to the summit were terrifying. I've lost count of how many times I've done the track since then.' He was packing up his stethoscope and other gear. 'Thanks for the offer of tea, Claire, but I'd better get going.' He glanced at the tray. 'That shortbread does look delicious.'

'Here…' Claire wrapped some biscuits in a paper serviette. 'Take some with you. It's Mum's family recipe and you might need some sustenance if you're going to be climbing the Pinnacles track.'

Colin Smythe picked Adam up from the front door of the Karaka Medical Centre fifteen minutes later, which had been just enough time for him to get back from Janet's house, grab his LandSAR gear from the back of his car and get into his overalls, jacket and heavy-duty hiking boots. He threw his pack into the back of the four-by-four and climbed into the back seat, because the front passenger seat was already occupied.

By Sam.

'Hey…' he greeted them both. 'Thanks for this.'

'Better to car pool,' Colin said. 'Keeps more space in the parking area for the other emergency vehicles or for a helicopter to land if necessary.'

'Any more details on what's happening?'

'Can you fill him in, Sam?' Colin asked. He was busy responding to a message on his phone.

'Sure.' Sam turned in her seat as Adam did up his safety belt. 'Lone tramper—a guy called Matty Savage who's a keen amateur photographer. He walked up to the Pinnacles Hut yesterday afternoon, spent the night in the hut and did the rest of the walk to the summit in time to get some sunrise shots. Other people at the summit said they saw him walking around getting photos but nobody saw him leave or on the track downhill.'

'There are two options,' Colin said, putting his phone down and starting up the engine. 'The Webb's Creek track via Hydro Camp, which is about halfway to the hut, or the Billygoat track. Longer and more challenging, with some river crossings.'

'Yep…' Adam was nodding. 'I know them both. Been up there a few times over the years.'

'The hut warden had checked him in and assigned him a bunk but he only had a day pack with him and was gone early. It's the friend he was supposed to meet for lunch who's raised the alarm. He drove up to the trailhead car park when Matty didn't turn up and he couldn't get him on the phone. His car's still there and he's now four hours overdue. His mate, Chris, is seriously concerned. He says it's really out of character. He's talked to everyone he's seen coming down and nobody's seen Matty on the main track. If someone's taken the longer track, they might still be on the way down.'

Sam twisted back to look at Adam again. 'You probably know these tracks better than either of us. What are your first thoughts?'

Oh, man…the way she was looking at him. As if what he was thinking and every word he was about to utter was important. To *her*.

It reminded him of the first time he'd been really captured by her gaze. At school that day, after his mother had invited Sam to dinner and Charlotte had been bouncing with excitement at the idea.

When he'd been totally under the spell of both acknowledging his physical attraction to this woman and soaking in the way she was looking at him, as if he was the person who could give her exactly what she wanted. More than that, even. That he could give her what she *needed*…

If that had been the first flicker of wanting to *be* that man, then what he was feeling right now was more like an out-of-control bushfire. If only he could be the one to give her the entire world and everything it could possibly offer.

Because he loved her. That much.

But he couldn't even tell her that. Because that shine in her eyes was there because she was doing what she loved the most right now. Throwing herself into the kind of search and rescue missions that were one of her passions. She knew what she wanted in life and she also knew what she didn't want.

Anchors.

People—or places—that might hold her back.

The only thing Adam *could* do was to give her the information she was asking for. It wasn't the first time he'd found himself by Sam's side in a situation like this but it was very likely to be the last and he wanted her to remember him as being, at the very least, a team member who would do anything he could to help her.

'I think that he's walking alone.' Adam found that he needed to clear his throat. 'That falls can happen, especially if you're distracted by something like trying to get the best shot, and that they can happen so fast they might not be seen by other people even if they're nearby.'

Colin's gaze was fixed on the road but he was nodding. 'What are your picks for the most dangerous spots, Adam? Those stone steps by Hydro Camp?'

'They can certainly get slippery,' Adam agreed. 'And it gets pretty steep around there. If he's gone via the Billy-goat, the river crossings can be dodgy if the water level's up but, for my money, the most likely place to fall and slip into a gully is around the summit. You're asking for trouble up there if you leave the track or ignore any fences.'

'That's what I said.' Sam sounded approving. 'How long will it take us to get to the summit?'

'It's a three-hour hike, if you're fit,' Colin said. 'But we've got a bit of work to do before we start walking.'

Sam was holding Adam's gaze and the gleam he saw in her eyes made him bite back a smile. He knew exactly how fit this woman was.

And dammit…he still wanted to be that person.

Her person.

He wanted it so much that he could actually feel a shaft of physical pain in his heart.

How bittersweet was this?

A collision of everything Samantha Gillespie could ever dream of having in her life.

She was in her happy place again, with her adventurous, thrill-seeking spirit being indulged just enough to keep it happy by the prospect of heading into wild country with a potentially injured person who needed both her technical and medical skills.

But there was another side to herself that she had only just realised hadn't been buried forever.

The part of her spirit that wanted nothing more than to love and be loved.

To have a family.

A place to call home.

How could one person be divided into what felt like complete opposites? It reminded Sam of how astonished she'd been that the chemistry between herself and Adam had been so explosively off the charts when they couldn't have been more different in their approaches to life.

It took another hour to get set up in the car parking area at the end of the road and assign roles to the increasing number of personnel arriving and Sam found herself stealing frequent glances at Adam as he helped her check the medical supplies and then they both listened to the planning and decisions being made between Colin and the police officer who was the search and rescue coordinator and in charge of this operation. They were discussing the logistics of the area and resources that might be needed in due course, like more searchers, rope experts to back up Tom, who was already here, handlers with dogs and possibly helicopters.

Standing a little outside the circle of people preparing to start the search was Chris, the friend of the missing person, Matty. He was currently watching a pair of trampers who were arriving back at the parking area and heading towards a rental car, staring back, open-mouthed, at the unusual activity in front of them.

'*Oi...*'

The loud sound from Chris made everyone turn. He was striding towards the man and his female companion.

'Where did you get that?' he shouted. 'That's Matty's.'

Both Adam and Sam turned sharply. Everybody else was watching them as they went to join Chris, who was now holding a black camera case in his hands.

'Are you absolutely sure it's Matty's?' Sam asked.

'Look.' Chris turned the case and she could see the sticker. A Baby Yoda, who was pointing to the words 'Light Side' and 'Dark Side' on either side of the switch above him. 'He's a hardcore Star Wars fan,' Chris said. 'This couldn't belong to anyone else.'

Colin had come over to them, closely followed by Tom and the police coordinator. 'Where did you find it?' he asked the couple.

'Up on the summit.' The man had an American accent. 'Looked like the wind had blown it over the edge of the cliff. I had to use a stick to get it but I thought someone might be missing it. We were going to leave it here, so they'd see it if they came back to look.'

'Did you see anything else?'

'I'm not sure, but I think there was something red further down the cliff. Couldn't say what it was. Bit of rubbish, maybe?'

Chris made a distressed sound. 'Matty was wearing a red jacket.'

'Okay…' Colin exchanged a look with Tom. 'We're going to need you to show us as best you can on a map, exactly where you found it.'

The new evidence and information completely changed the atmosphere of this pre-deployment gathering because it not only gave them the most likely point to start the search, it seemed very likely that the missing person was going to be badly injured. If he was still alive. Suddenly, things were urgent and taking three hours or more to get to the summit on foot was not an acceptable option. A helicopter was needed to ferry people up to the landing pad beside the hut but nothing was available immediately from the emergency services. A LandSAR volunteer had a local contact, however, who did heli-tourism and hunting trips and was on call to help if needed and they were on scene with admirable speed.

Sam was on the same trip up as Adam. Colin and Tom, with his climbing equipment, also managed to squeeze into the Squirrel helicopter despite the amount of gear they'd already put on board. With no air rescue medical crew available yet, the doctors' skills and kits might be the most needed if they could get close to their target.

Looking out of the window, Sam could see Chris watching them take off, his face a mask of fear. Turning her head, she could see Adam's expression. He looked serious and there were lines of tension deepening the crinkles around his eyes, but they were all feeling that. Nobody knew how much time, if any, they had left to save a life. But this was Adam's first mission. Was he nervous? Regretting his choices because he could be potentially putting himself in danger?

As if he felt her looking at him, Adam shifted his gaze from the window and Sam felt any concern evaporating.

She could see that Adam was more than comfortable with the choices he'd made and where he was right now. Unlike the day Sam had first met him in a very similar car park setting to the one they'd just taken off from. He'd been determined enough that day, mind you—he'd just been a long way out of his comfort zone. Or had fear threatened to overwhelm him because his precious daughter was one of the children who were trapped by the flooded creek?

Yeah…that had been one of her very first impressions, hadn't it? That this man would do whatever it took to protect Charlotte.

But here he was in a helicopter, heading towards the unknown, and Sam was sure she saw a hint of a smile curling one side of his mouth as he broke the eye contact to look out of the window again. The chopper had lifted high enough to start going forward and it was tilting to swoop over the swing bridge that crossed the river, gaining more height as the pilot followed the track that vanished into the lush bush-clad slopes beneath them. Was Adam feeling the same kind of adrenaline rush that Sam always did at a time like this?

Did he have a well-hidden *wild* side?

Was that why they felt like such a perfect fit? Because

they each embodied exactly what was missing from the other's life?

Yin and Yang.

Not that Adam would have been likely to acknowledge that. Or maybe he had and that had been enough to scare him into jumping at the opportunity to escape.

Whatever.

Perhaps they had touched each other's lives in ways that meant they would never forget each other. Sam hoped that Adam would keep up his connection to search and rescue work after she was gone. She knew perfectly well that she would never again experience what it was like to make love rather than simply have sex, but at least that was a choice *she* was making. Her life wasn't about to be up-ended by having it ripped away from her. And Adam was, no doubt, busy repairing any damage she might have done to his safety barriers, whether he was aware of it or not.

It was still a few hours before daylight would really start to fade at this time of year and as they got over the roofs of the hut buildings the pilot took them further, to hover over the jagged protrusions of what was left of an ancient volcano and the steep rocky slopes that lay beneath them. And they could all see the flash of colour that was a good ten metres from the top and probably hidden by a ledge from anyone looking down from above. The colour was red. The colour of Matty's jacket.

'Target sighted,' the pilot said.

'No sign of movement.' Colin's voice was grim.

Without conscious thought, Sam crossed her fingers inside her gloves. She very much wanted this mission to be successful. That they would find their missing person alive and be able to get him out to safety.

It might still be a bittersweet memory but, in a way, it could be the perfect ending to a part of her life that Sam would not have wanted to miss. She and Adam had come full circle. Back to where they'd started. Both different people but…maybe they both knew themselves a little better and that would change their lives for the better going forward.

Sam certainly felt older and wiser.

Getting to the summit as quickly as possible was a challenge, given the steep ascent with countless steps, ladders, tree roots and boulders to scramble over and the heavy packs of gear they needed to carry. There was no chance to pause and take in the astonishing views over the mountains to the coast and very little energy left for talking. With the helicopter returning to the car park to load the next group of SAR personnel, all Adam could hear was the crunch of his boots on the track and the huff of his heavy breathing.

Tom put ropes on the packs and hauled them up the steepest sections while Adam and Sam climbed the ladders and rocks with their metal rungs unencumbered. They didn't go as far as the wooden viewing platform right at the top.

'That's it.' Colin was pointing at a group of tall pointed rocks to one side of the track. 'That's where the camera bag was found.' He moved carefully off the track to peer down the slope. 'I can't see anything red. Could be he's moved further under that ledge.'

Adam and Sam exchanged a glance. If he'd moved since being first spotted, it could mean he was still alive. Sam unclipped a helmet from the side of her pack and put it on. Then she stepped into a climbing harness.

'Those rock spires look like excellent anchors,' Tom

said, sliding a long coil of rope from his shoulder. 'What do you think, Sam?'

'Couldn't be better,' Sam agreed. 'Adam—could you please get as much as you can into the small trauma pack? Just the essentials to start with—airway kit, pressure dressings, CAT tourniquet, haemostatic gauze. A SAM splint and some pain relief. Intranasal fentanyl and ketamine. And the IV kit, please.' She was buckling up her harness. 'Anything else can be lowered down in one of the bigger packs by rope. Tom and Colin will sort that.'

'You'll need help,' Adam said. 'Is there a way I can get down?'

'Have you ever done any abseiling?'

'No.'

'Then no,' Sam said decisively. 'Too dangerous.' She tightened the chin strap of her helmet. 'If he's still alive, we'll get backup on the way. He'd have to be winched out, anyway. There's no way we'd get a stretcher back up this cliff.'

Once the manageably sized trauma kit was sorted, there was nothing for Adam to do other than stand and watch as Tom, Colin and the next wave of the rescue team arrived and went into action. Adam knew very little about abseiling but he could see that great care was being taken to attach ropes to the spikes of rock at the top and there seemed to be a huge number of carabiners and other pieces of equipment that were checked and double-checked before Sam began attaching them to her harness.

She looked like a total professional in all her gear and helmet and gloves, leaning back over the edge of the cliff and testing her radio comms before she started her descent.

She looked calm, confident and...unbelievably sexy. Every inch the superhero that Charlotte thought Dr Sam was.

Adam's heart was in his mouth as he saw Sam leaning even further out and taking what looked like a leap into space as she released some of the rope in her hands. He could imagine Charlotte watching this with wide eyes and hands clasped in awe. Would he want her to have a role model that might inspire her to do something like this in the future?

Yes—if it had all the checks and balances for safety that an organisation like LandSAR had in place. But Sam as her role model? If she knew what *he* knew about her? He could live with the thought that Charlotte might end up thinking it would be cool to get into abseiling as a hobby, but what if she decided it might be cool to try something as dangerous as roof topping? That was...unthinkable.

Perhaps he should be grateful that his daughter was never going to get the chance to know Sam as well as he did. And wasn't that the reason he'd decided it was safe to get close to Sam in the first place? Because she didn't want to stick around any more than she wanted a relationship? This was always how it had been going to end. It was entirely appropriate that it was finishing with this kind of dramatic flourish, in fact.

A helicopter was hovering overhead now. It was the same one that had brought him and Sam up here but there were no LandSAR people in the back this time. The side door was open and Adam could see someone with a big camera pointed towards them all. Had a television news crew been deployed this fast?

The break in his focus on Sam had only been for a heartbeat but something had changed as he looked back to where she was, several metres down now, navigating her way past an outcrop of small boulders, one of which came loose under her foot and rolled free to bounce down the cliff.

Colin made a growling sound. 'Be careful, Sam,' Adam heard him mutter. 'That section's unstable.'

The beat of fear his words invoked should have reinforced any thoughts that Charlotte might be safer by not having Sam as a role model as she grew up but, oddly, it had the opposite effect. He could feel Sam's focus even from this far away. Her determination. Her courage.

He knew how much she cared about what she did in life. How much she could care about people and...

And that was exactly the kind of person he hoped that Charlotte would grow up to be like. Someone who was passionate about life. Someone fierce and independent and fearless.

Someone *exactly* like Sam.

She had half his genes, after all, and surely that would provide balance. The best of both worlds. Courage with a dollop of caution. Risk-taking—with a safety net, like his part in this rescue team—but rewards that would be more meaningful because of that element of risk.

Sam was well down the cliff now, almost at the ledge.

And then it happened.

Another boulder, even bigger than the first one, was coming loose from the unstable section and starting to move. A shower of earth was a warning that it had reached a tipping point and there was a chorus of shouts from everybody around Adam.

'*Sam*... Look *out*...'

Adam saw her head flick up and knew that she could see the huge rock coming towards her. He saw her plant her feet against the cliff and push out, swinging away from the path of the missile. He saw the rope jerk as it got brushed and then the way Sam swung back in, out of control now, to slam against the rockface.

Maybe he was imagining it, but in that split second where he could almost feel the impact of that unforgiving rock wall against Sam's body, he was sure he could also hear the sound of her cry cutting through the roar of the helicopter rotors so close overhead he could feel his own body bracing against the powerful downwash of air.

The bracing wasn't a conscious action. In that moment it felt as if he'd been turned to stone. Completely frozen. Spun back in time. He had lost his footing and his balance and any control over anything that was happening around him.

There was only one thing he could be absolutely sure about.

He'd been right.

Falling in love with anyone was a mistake he should never have made.

And falling in love with Samantha Gillespie was the biggest version of that mistake he could have made. His heart was splitting open, knowing that he had probably just lost her far more definitively than by her simply moving to another city, and the pain coming towards him like a tsunami was inescapable.

There was only one thing he could hang onto. The same thing he'd been hanging onto ever since this had all begun. It had to be enough, even facing what felt like an unbearable loss.

Adam had at least managed to protect Charlotte.

Colin was on his radio.

'Sam… *Sam*… Can you hear me?'

CHAPTER ELEVEN

THE IMPACT WINDED HER.

There was such a loud ringing in Sam's ears that the sound of her name felt as if someone was shouting from a huge distance.

'Sam… *Sam…*'

She was still fighting to get a breath. Clinging to a protrusion in the rock wall in front of her face with both her gloved hands. Blinking to try and clear her vision. Had she been knocked out and was only now regaining consciousness? No…she could remember everything. Seeing that boulder coming directly towards her. Pushing with all her strength to try and get out of its trajectory. She'd almost felt the brush of that rock as it passed by so closely and she'd definitely been aware of the spinning that shouldn't have happened and then the impact of hitting the cliff.

She'd hadn't been knocked out because she could also remember groping for any hand-hold she could find to support herself against the wall and keep some weight out of her harness until she could check her gear and both her main and backup ropes. She was still holding tight to rock. She'd even found enough of a ledge for her toes to press into so she was in contact with the cliff with all her limbs, hanging there like a human spider.

It had been a very close call, but Sam couldn't afford to think about just how close it *had* been. That would, no doubt, come back to haunt her later, but it wouldn't help anyone to go there now. She allowed herself a heartbeat to realise how astonishingly lucky she'd been and then move on. She needed to make sure she had only been winded by the impact and then move on with what she was supposed to be doing.

She couldn't feel any pain anywhere in her body and her muscles were responding to the lightning-fast, head-to-toe check she gave them. She knew she'd bumped her head hard enough to make her ears ring but she was quite confident that her helmet had protected her. The rim, or perhaps some debris, had dug into her forehead with enough force to break the skin, though, because she re-alised it was blood trickling into her eye.

She blinked again as she cautiously reached for her radio.

'I'm okay,' she said. 'What happened?'

'Rockfall.' Colin's voice was grim. 'Made contact with your rope and sent you into a spin. Are you sure you're not hurt?'

'Just winded for a sec. Okay now.'

'Have you got an anchor you can use while we check the ropes?'

Sam looked around her. An exposed tree root coming from between rocks looked promising. She grasped it with her hand and gave it some steady, increasing pressure. It felt as solid as the rock it was embedded in.

'Yes. Am connecting my cow's tail so I can check the rope.'

Sam slipped the short length of rope clipped to her harness around the tree root and secured it. Then she looked up at her rope to see if any damage like fraying or flattening was visible. It wasn't. She pushed the button on her radio again.

'Sam to Tom. Do you read?'

'Roger.'

'Can you see any damage?'

'No.'

Sam looked down. She was less than a few metres to the sloping base of this gully. Twisting her head, she could see more of the red fabric of that jacket. She could see that there was a person inside it now.

'Matty?' she called. 'Can you hear me?'

She couldn't hear a response. But she could see a hand lifting and that was enough.

'Don't move,' she shouted. 'I'm on my way.'

There was no relief from the roller coaster that Adam had inadvertently climbed aboard.

He'd been fine with the adrenaline rush of the helicopter ride up into the mountains and the more hair-raising sections of the scramble to the summit. He'd been prepared to watch Sam calmly putting herself in danger to be the one to get to their patient first. She was, after all, the only person qualified to both rappel down a cliff face and then provide the medical care a badly injured person would need. She might be putting herself at risk but she was doing it with all the safety checks and balances that were available.

He hadn't been prepared for the shock of seeing Sam almost being taken out by a falling boulder, but what had made him hit rock-bottom with such a crunch had been to realise the effect that losing her would have. On *him*. He could feel the weight of the kind of grief that was so deep it never really left. Just for a second or two, before the relief of hearing her voice over the radio had been enough to have him blinking back tears, but nothing was ever going to be the same. The reminder of exactly why getting involved with anyone had been off the table for the last five years had hit him with a vengeance. How had he thought it was safe, simply because he knew it wasn't going to last?

He couldn't find anything safe to hang onto right now, so he needed to distance himself somehow. To gather resources he wasn't that sure that he even had available, because he still had no idea when—or how—this emotional ride was really going to end. He listened to the radio exchanges between Sam and Colin and then Sam and Tom as she checked her ropes and then decided to finish her descent.

'Matty's alive,' he heard her say, as if nothing else mattered. 'I'm going down.'

He listened to her first, slightly breathless report after what felt like an interminable silence as she presumably did a primary and then secondary survey to assess their patient.

'Airway's clear but breathing's rapid, shallow and painful. Tachycardic at one twenty but BP currently one ten over seventy. He thinks he got knocked out. No signs of skull fracture and pupils equal and reactive, but he's got a moderate concussion with repetitive speech and confusion—GCS fourteen. He's got multiple fractures to his ribs, left arm and right tib/fib. Also left upper quadrant abdominal pain—query spleen, and I can't rule out a spinal injury. I'll give him some pain relief, try to splint his arm and keep him as immobile and warm as possible, but we need evacuation ASAP.'

'On its way already,' Colin told her. 'ETA is ten minutes.'

A professional focus on the young man who'd fallen was helpful now. It was amazing he was still alive after that fall, but his injuries were concerning and things could take a turn for the worse at any moment. A broken rib could have punctured a lung or blood vessel and be affecting his breathing by more than causing pain. If his spleen had ruptured, he could be losing enough blood to tip him into hypovolaemic shock. He might have a head injury that was a lot more serious than concussion and an undiagnosed spinal injury could mean the risk of paralysis if he moved before being properly immobilised with a rigid neck collar and a vacuum mattress for the rest of his body.

Yes…this was definitely helping. The professional arena was generating a distance between himself and Sam. Adam knew perfectly well that it wouldn't last but, for now, he was grateful.

He held his breath as the rescue helicopter hovered overhead, the one with the cameramen on board now at a safe distance but clearly still filming the drama. A paramedic was winched down and Sam worked with them to package Matty so that he could be winched back up to the chopper.

'What's going to happen for Sam?' he asked Colin. 'Does she have to climb back up the cliff?'

He shook his head. 'That's not an option, even if we replace her ropes. Not when there's a real risk there are more loose rocks. They'll send someone down to winch her up to the chopper and I imagine they'll touch down on the pad at the hut to let her off.'

Adam waited only until he'd seen Sam pulled safely into the cabin of the helicopter before he joined the others to start the descent back to the hut. It was faster going downhill but he had to be careful not to get too fast. The last thing he wanted was to slip on a ladder or staircase and create another patient for the LandSAR team to have to rescue. As the minutes ticked past and he strode swiftly along a flatter part of the track, it occurred to him to wonder why he hadn't seen the bright red helicopter lifting off again to head for the nearest major hospital's emergency department.

He found out as he got close enough to see that the helicopter was still on the landing pad near the hut. The doors were open and he could also see that Sam was still inside with the crew. He increased his pace to get even closer but Colin's voice made him pause.

'*Whoa*…where are you going, Adam?'

'They must have a medical complication to deal with. I was going to see if they need any more assistance.'

'Fair enough, but you don't just approach a helicopter that's hot loading.'

Adam nodded. He'd done a session on safety around helicopters in his training already. 'I know to stay crouched,' he said. 'And only approach from the front or side, where the pilot can see me.'

'You also need permission from the pilot.' Colin lifted his radio. 'It's a confined space. They may not need anyone else in there.'

Adam had to bite back the words that wanted to emerge.

But what about Sam? What if she needs me?

And then it hit him. Why *would* she need him? She had the experts in pre-hospital and retrieval medicine inside that helicopter with her. Her future colleagues. The only thing he could do was to cheer her on from the sidelines—as a friend. He had no further part to play in this scenario. Maybe this was a timely reminder that he had no further part to play in the new life that Sam was about to embark on.

It seemed that Adam had finally reached the end of that roller coaster ride and he could climb, albeit shakily, out of the car. A welcome numbing effect was happening to cushion the effects of the emotional wringer he'd just been through.

He watched Sam climbing out of the side door of the aircraft a short time later and it closed behind her straight away. She kept her head low and moved swiftly to get clear and, just as quickly, the helicopter lifted off and headed back towards the mountains and the cities beyond this peninsula.

She pulled her helmet off as she got closer to Adam and he was horrified to see the cut on the side of her forehead and the remnants of dried blood on her skin that was the palest he'd ever seen it. He could also see that she'd been holding things together in order to do her job, which was no surprise, but that perhaps the shock of having almost been killed was finally hitting her. He could sense how rigidly she was holding herself, almost visibly trembling with the effort.

This was no time to remind her that she was facing that kind of risk every time she threw herself into situations like this. Or that it affected other people as well as herself. Good grief, if he said anything like that, he might find himself confessing how much it had affected *him*. That he might have known he was in love with her but he'd only just realised that telling himself he could cope with not having her in his life—that it might even be a good thing that she was moving on—had been no more than a smokescreen, or perhaps a safety barrier he hadn't noticed was already crumbling. *Really* not having her in his life, at all, was going to be the hardest thing he'd faced since the day he'd greeted his newborn daughter and had to say goodbye to her mother.

No. He couldn't say any of that. He knew Sam had been given just as much, if not more, of a fright as he had. The last thing she needed was for him to make it any more difficult to try and get her head straight. He had to fight the urge to hold out his arms and invite her into them and hold her as tightly as he would if he had no intention of ever letting her go. Holding Sam that close might well reveal far more than either of them would find comfortable and it certainly wouldn't help his chances of repairing boundaries. The ones that could keep both him and Charlotte safe in the future.

So he barely met her gaze as he shook his head slowly.

'Oh, my God, Sam,' was all he murmured.

'Close call,' she agreed. 'Matty developed a tension pneumothorax thanks to his broken ribs. I got winched up just as he went into respiratory arrest. That's why we were on the ground for so long here. I ended up doing a finger thoracotomy. Hopefully, the guys will get him into Theatre before any other deterioration.'

'He's lucky to still be alive.'

'Yeah…' The note in Sam's voice said it all. She was just as lucky.

'You okay?' Colin's voice was gruff. He was the one who wrapped Sam in a rough hug and squeezed her. 'You gave us all one hell of a fright, Sam.'

'I'm fine.'

Adam could sense the way Sam was trying to pull herself together and put on a brave face now. It also felt like she might be avoiding looking at him.

'You know what they say,' she added, a brightness in her voice that didn't ring true. 'A miss is as good as a mile. I've just got a few bumps and bruises.'

'And that cut on your head,' Adam growled. 'I'll clean that up for you.'

Some of the group opted to walk down the track back to the car park but the others, including Adam and Sam, went into the hut to wait for the local helicopter to come back for them. A three-hour trek would mean it would be well past sunset by the time they got back to their vehicles.

Adam didn't say a word as he gently swabbed the wound with some gauze soaked in saline and disinfectant. Neither did Sam.

He suspected that was partly due to exhaustion but that the main reason was more likely to be that there was nothing to say. Not when other people might overhear it, anyway.

He dried the skin thoroughly. 'We don't have skin glue anywhere in the kit, do we?'

'No. There's Steri-Strips.'

'They'll do. You might be left with a bit of a scar, though. And a black eye. The bruising's coming up already.' Adam's light touch on the skin close to the corner of Sam's eye was not entirely clinical.

The way he held Sam's gaze wasn't either.

'This could have been so much worse,' he said, unable to cover the crack in his voice. 'I thought it *was* so much worse.'

She knew. He could see the empathy in her eyes. The apology that he'd been reminded of loss. A frisson of the connection they had in knowing how hard it was to lose someone you loved.

'I'm sorry,' she murmured. 'But all's well that ends well, isn't it? I hope you won't let what happened with me put you off.'

What was that supposed to mean? Not to let the close call put him off doing rescue work? Or was it a suggestion that he didn't need to be put off having a relationship with someone, as long as it wasn't with *her*?

The look in her eyes told him it might be both. The wry smile told him that this was what they'd known all along. That they were too different.

That it could never have worked.

That perhaps they could count themselves lucky they were escaping relatively unscathed—from both what had happened today and what could have happened if they hadn't agreed it was time to stop seeing each other.

And maybe that was that.

This really was the end.

Adam pulled the edges of the cut together with the super-sticky strips. 'Try and keep it clean and dry,' he said, his tone neutral. 'See a doctor if there are any signs of infection.'

The hint of a wry smile curled one corner of Sam's mouth. 'Will do.'

'Have you got a headache?'

'No.'

Adam shone a pen torch into her eyes and then clipped it back onto his pocket and put his hands over her scalp, gently palpating for any injuries that might be hidden by her hair.

'Anything hurt?'

'No.'

He held her head in both his hands, moving it carefully. 'Any neck pain?'

'No.'

'Good.'

It *was* good. It meant that Adam could take his hands away from her skin. From her warmth and scent and memories of touching her in very, very different circumstances. They could all hear the sound of a helicopter landing nearby so it was time to get back to the helipad. Back to their normal lives, even though Adam had a feeling his life was never going to be quite the same after this.

'Call me,' he told Sam, 'if you feel unwell in any way later tonight. Or...' He hesitated. What had he been about to say? Or if there was anything else he could do for her? Or if she wanted to talk about the fright she'd had? Or if she simply wanted some company?

His mind snuck in another query. What about *you*? What is it that *you* want?

Adam knew the answer to that instantly. He wanted to get back to his safe space. His home. And his family.

Maybe Sam had also known the answer to that question.

'I'll be fine, Adam,' she said as she got to her feet. 'I always am. Don't worry about me.'

That feeling that his life had been irrevocably changed in the last few hours got even stronger as Adam walked up the path to his front door.

It spiked even higher when the door opened before he'd been able to put his key in the lock.

'*Adam…*' Jude Carter sounded beyond relieved. 'Thank *goodness* you're home.'

'What's wrong?' His question was almost a bark as he stepped through the door. 'Is it Charlie?'

His mother's face scrunched into distressed lines. 'It was my fault,' she said. 'I put the news on television. I thought that maybe they'd mention whether you'd been successful in the search you were doing but…'

'But *what*?' Adam was striding down the hallway now.

'They were filming everything. Charlie thought it might be Sam climbing down the cliff and she was glued to the screen.'

'It *was* Sam,' Adam said, throwing a glance over his shoulder.

'Oh, no…' Jude had her hand to her mouth. 'She saw the accident. That big rock falling and the way she hit the cliff. She's been beside herself ever since.'

Adam could hear the exhausted sobbing as he reached the door of Charlotte's bedroom. His daughter was curled into a surprisingly small ball on her bed but she lifted her face at the sound of voices and when she saw her father she lifted her arms, her whimper a piteous sound of pain.

He scooped her up and sat on the bed with Charlotte on his lap, folded into his arms.

'It's okay,' he said over and over again as he stroked her hair. 'It's okay, peanut. Everything's okay…'

Except it wasn't, was it?

He could feel Charlotte shaking—like Sam had been when the adrenaline was wearing off after her fright, but this was worse. This was a small, vulnerable child who hadn't chosen to put herself in harm's way but she'd been hurt anyway.

'The only person who got hurt was the man who was being rescued,' he added.

'I told her that.' Jude sounded as if she was struggling to hold back tears herself. 'They said it on the news. Nobody was injured and the person who fell is in a serious but stable condition in hospital.'

Adam pressed a kiss into Charlotte's hair and kept his cheek against her head, speaking as reassuringly as he could. 'Dr Sam is fine. She got a bit of a bump but she still went and looked after the man who fell down the cliff. Because she's a superhero, isn't she?'

But Charlotte shook her head. 'She got hurt. I saw it. I thought she was…*dead*. Like Mummy…'

Oh, dear *Lord*…

Adam knew that Charlotte couldn't possibly have any real memories of her mother. Or of losing her. But this felt as if she knew exactly what his own grief had been like. His big-hearted little girl, who cared so much about the people she loved, was distraught. He remembered the way she'd initially refused to get rescued, that day they'd both met Sam, because she had to sit beside her beloved teacher and hold her hand to comfort her. That little heart was breaking now and he had no idea how to make it better.

'Dr Sam just got a little ouchie on her head, that's all.' He tried to sound like it was no big deal. 'I put a plaster on it. Like I do on your ouchies. She's fine, I promise…'

But Charlotte shook her head, her nose rubbing on Adam's collarbone. 'I don't believe you,' she wailed. 'I'm never going to see Dr Sam again, am I?'

Okay… That desperate need to offer comfort and re-assurance was getting laced with another emotion that Adam wasn't about to encourage by dwelling on it. It might be that his daughter's pain was contagious. Or it could be that he was starting to feel angry that she was experiencing it at all.

This was why he'd never wanted to risk having some-one else in his life. Until he'd met Sam. And the one person who could have made him break through those boundaries had been someone who spent her life looking for opportunities to hurl herself into danger. How *stupid* had he been?

It might even get worse. In a few days from now, Samantha Gillespie would be leaving town and it could turn out to be true that Charlotte would never see her again.

At least he knew what he had to do right now. He stood up, with Charlotte still sobbing in his arms.

'I can fix this,' he told his mother. 'There's only one way to make her believe that Sam's okay.' He was walking towards the front door. 'We'll be back soon.'

CHAPTER TWELVE

TIRED BUT WIRED.

A catchphrase that was a common response amongst emergency service personnel when asked how they were doing in the aftermath of a stressful event, but it seemed too flippant to cover how Sam was feeling when she was finally home, in the peace and quiet of her half of the old house that she rented.

The flood of adrenaline that had been released in a moment of extreme danger had kept her going long enough to do what she had to do after surviving that near miss—to assess Matty and care for him until backup arrived. But then, it had been Matty who'd nearly died when he suffered a respiratory arrest and the invasive procedure Sam had performed to make a hole in the side of his chest and release the pressure of the blood and air that had stopped him breathing had sucked up even more of the autonomic response of her body to either fight, take flight or freeze when facing danger.

Was feeling like this on a regular basis really her dream career?

Right now, she was less sure about that. But she wasn't sure about anything, was she? She didn't quite know what to think. Or what to do with herself.

She wouldn't be able to eat anything for hours. Blood flow had been redirected from her stomach and digestive system to her muscles and just the thought of food made her feel sick.

She had a wild desire to pull off her overalls and boots and put on some leggings and trainers and run, but it was almost dark outside and the concept of 'tiredness' was nothing like the level of exhaustion that had taken over her muscles to the extent that pulling in air to fill her lungs felt like an effort.

Why couldn't her brain have the same lack of energy or motivation? If anything, it was going faster than normal, darting from one image or movie reel to another. Letting her experience the sensation of one emotion and then another and randomly throwing in things from the past just for a bit of extra spice.

Sam was pacing, stopping occasionally to stare at something that made no impression on her, like the cushions on her couch or crumbs that needed cleaning off her kitchen bench.

What she was actually seeing was a flashback to that massive lump of rock hurtling towards her and feeling the dread that it might very well be the last thing she ever saw.

Seeing her fingers shake, just for a nanosecond, before she pushed the tip of the scalpel into the skin of Matty's chest between his ribs and feeling the pressure of knowing that this young man would die very quickly if she couldn't do this procedure correctly and swiftly enough.

Seeing the way Adam's gaze had slid away from her own, as if he didn't want the intimacy of eye contact, let alone the physical contact of giving her a hug. Feeling bereft because a hug was what she'd needed the most right then. To be held tightly enough to believe that everything was going to be okay.

But he hadn't wanted to, and she understood that. This was why she could never let people into the core of her life. Thank goodness they'd managed to stop themselves getting into a real relationship with each other. Imagine if she'd been responsible for Adam having to lose another person that he was in a significant relationship with. If he'd had to relive that kind of trauma, even though it would have only been an echo of what he'd gone through in losing the woman he'd loved enough to marry. The mother of his precious child…

No. It didn't feel like anything was going to be okay any time soon, but Sam had no idea what to do to try and make it better. So she kept pacing.

Until she heard the knock on her door.

A loud knock. Demanding. Angry?

When Sam opened her door to find Adam outside, with Charlotte in his arms, he wasn't avoiding eye contact this time. Quite the opposite. He was holding hers with a stare that meant *she* couldn't look away.

Yeah…he was angry.

And Sam knew why the moment Charlotte raised her tear-stained face from where it had been buried against her father's shoulder.

'Dr Sam,' she sobbed, 'I thought you were *dead*…'

Charlotte somehow managed to throw herself from her father's arms, wrapping her arms around Sam's neck and her legs around her waist, clinging to her like a monkey. It was an automatic response to put her own arms around this child to keep her safe and then it was impossible not to hold her even closer. To press her face against the soft, dark hair that was unravelling itself from its usual braids.

'Of course I'm not dead, sweetheart,' she said. 'Whatever made you think that?'

'She saw you.' Adam's voice was controlled. Cool. So cool the words sounded as if they were coated with a film of ice. 'On the news. They managed to capture every moment of that rockfall.'

Oh, *no…*

The knowledge that she had scared Charlotte was heartbreaking.

The feeling of holding this little girl in her arms was also heartbreaking. She could feel Charlotte's heart against her own ribs, going too fast in a small chest that was still heaving with sobs that were only starting to subside. How long had she been crying like this? What sort of nightmares might she have tonight?

Sam felt guilty as well as heartbroken now. She totally deserved the anger being directed at her via Adam's stare. She had failed to maintain her distance from other people enough to protect them from her own actions. She'd never intended to let that happen. She knew how badly it could affect other people if they cared too much. Even now, she could still feel what it had been like to hold Robbie in her arms as he took his last breath.

Charlotte was staring up at her. She caught her breath in a hiccup that signalled the end of her misery and then she reached up to touch Sam's face.

'You got an ouchie,' she said. 'Does it still hurt?'

*Oh…*the caring in Charlotte's voice. The soft touch of those small fingers. The love in those big brown eyes.

'No, it doesn't hurt, sweetheart,' she said softly. 'It's just a scratch, but I'll be more careful next time, I promise.'

Charlotte was smiling at her. 'That's what Daddy always says when I get an ouchie. He says "Be more careful next time, won't you, Charlie?".'

There was a tiny sparkle in her eyes now. A gleam of mischief, even—as if she was sharing the secret that she might not be that careful next time but it didn't matter because she was safe in the knowledge that her daddy would be there to make any ouchie better. It gave Sam the same kind of internal squeeze that being in their home had generated, of a place filled with love. A real home. A real family.

If her heart had already been cracked open by knowing she'd hurt Charlotte by scaring her, it was shattering into thousands of pieces now.

Because Sam was aware of something else that was going to break her heart forever.

She'd never held a child like this before. Ever. She'd dealt with any number of children as a doctor and even held them sometimes, but this was so very different. This was a child who had not only captured Sam's heart, she'd given her own without hesitation. She was such an adorable child and Sam loved her as wholeheartedly as she loved her father.

How horrified would Adam be if he knew that? Charlotte had no idea of how close she and Adam had become but look at how miserable Sam's actions had made her today. She could understand completely how Adam wasn't prepared to risk his daughter's happiness by letting her get really attached to someone. And Sam cared about them both too much to try and push her way any closer. Even if she desperately wanted to.

But Sam knew now, without a shadow of doubt, that the thing she could never have was what she wanted more than anything else in life.

A family of her own.

As if he could sense what she was thinking, or rather simply feeling with every cell in her body, Adam reached out and peeled Charlotte away from her.

'See?' he asked, smiling as he pulled his daughter into his own arms. 'I told you that Dr Sam was okay. It's time for us to go home now. Okay?'

'Okay, Daddy.' Charlotte was snuggling in closer. Her eyes were drifting shut as the exhaustion of overwhelming emotions caught up with her.

Sam knew how she felt.

She watched Adam tuck her into her car seat and close the door. He was about to walk around to the driver's door but, instead, he swerved and strode back towards where she was still standing in the open door.

His words were a low growl that Charlotte wouldn't have heard even if she was still awake.

'I was dreading you leaving,' he said. 'But, you know what?' He didn't give her a chance to respond to the question. He did it himself. 'I think it's the only way of fixing this. The sooner it's over, the better.'

Sam pushed her front door closed as he turned back to his car because she couldn't bear to watch him walk away. Then she rested her head against it until she heard the car pulling away and the sound of the engine fading into silence.

Even then, she couldn't move.

Not even to brush away the tears that were rolling down her face.

* * *

Charlotte was sound asleep by the time Adam got back home.

His mother had been watching out for them and she opened the door as he came up the steps. He paused long enough for Jude to stroke back some wisps of hair from Charlotte's face and smile at her granddaughter.

'She looks so peaceful. It would be a shame to wake her up for her dinner.'

'Let's not,' Adam agreed. 'I'll tuck her into bed. I think she needs her sleep more than food.'

Jude followed them down the hallway. 'I'm so sorry, Adam. It was my fault. I shouldn't have had the television on.'

'You didn't know what was about to happen,' Adam reminded her. 'None of us did. If anything, it was my fault for being there. You wouldn't have known what was going on and turned the news on in the first place if I hadn't signed up for LandSAR.'

'I was so proud, knowing you were there,' Jude said. 'But poor Sam…it must have given her an awful fright.' She was shaking her head as she passed Charlotte's bedroom door on her way back to the kitchen. 'I think she's the bravest woman I've ever met.'

Adam's response was no more than a grunt. He carried Charlotte into her room and carefully peeled away her shoes and clothes. She roused enough to push her arms into the sleeves of her pyjamas and then reached for her fluffy red panda toy to clutch in her arms as her head hit the pillow. When Adam bent down to give her a goodnight kiss, however, her eyes opened again.

'Don't go, Daddy.'

'Okay. I'll stay here until you're asleep again. Do you want me to get you a snack?'

Charlotte shook her head. 'I'm not hungry.'

Adam sat on her bed and leaned against the wall. 'But you feel better now?' he asked. 'Now that you know that Dr Sam is really okay?'

Charlotte nodded this time, her eyes drifting shut and a smile tilting her lips. Adam waited, watching for her breathing to slow and to hear those cute snuffly sounds that were a sure sign that she was properly asleep, but suddenly her eyes popped open again.

'Do you know what, Daddy?'

'What?'

'If I could pick any mummy in the whole world, do you know who I'd pick?'

'Um… Gamma?'

'*No…*' The word was a fond dismissal. 'Don't be silly, Daddy. She's my gamma.'

'Oh…is it Miss Kempsey?'

'No…' This time Charlotte giggled. 'She's my *teacher.*'

It was Adam's turn to close his eyes. He knew what was coming. He knew what his next guess had to be, but he couldn't bring himself to say the name.

So Charlotte did it for him.

'Dr Sam,' she said. 'I love Dr Sam *so* much.'

'So do I, button.' The words slipped out without any hesitation. As if they'd been waiting for the opportunity to emerge.

There was a beat of silence. The only light in the room came from Charlotte's night light that was a magic mushroom with tiny fairies dancing around the stalk. Charlotte's voice, when she broke the silence, was thoughtful.

'So if *you* love her and *I* love her, why *can't* she be my mummy?'

'She would have to feel the same way,' Adam pointed out.

'How do you know she doesn't?'

'I don't,' he had to admit.

'So can you ask her? Tomorrow?'

Oh, *help*. How did he go about trying to explain why this couldn't happen? He'd always been as open with Charlotte as she was capable of understanding and had never hesitated to make it feel as though her mother still had a place in their lives, but this was a whole new ballgame. If he brushed a response off because it was difficult, would that make Charlotte less likely to be open with him as she grew up? Adam didn't want that to happen.

'You remember how sad you were when you saw the news tonight and you thought that Sam had been hurt?'

Charlotte hugged her panda closer. 'I thought she was dead,' she said in a dramatic whisper. 'Like my first mummy.'

'And you were really sad, weren't you?'

Charlotte nodded.

'Well, maybe Sam thinks she can't be someone's mummy because she doesn't want to make them sad.'

'Why?'

'Well...' Adam reached out to stroke Charlotte's hair. 'Nobody wants the people they love to be sad, do they?'

Charlotte's brow furrowed. 'No... I meant why would she make someone sad?'

'Because she does things that can be dangerous and sometimes accidents happen—like today—so it's possible she could get hurt.'

'But she didn't get hurt. She just got an ouchie. I get ouchies all the time.'

'She didn't get hurt this time,' Adam agreed.

'Maybe she won't ever get hurt. She promised to be really careful next time.'

'But accidents can happen,' Adam said carefully. 'Sam loves doing things that can be dangerous and she wouldn't want to stop doing them because it might make other people sad.'

Charlotte was wide awake now and looking totally confused. Adam's heart sank. He was not doing a good job of explaining this, was he?

'Why would she want to stop?' Charlotte asked. 'She's Dr Sam. That's what she *does*.'

That was true. It wasn't just what Sam did. It was who she was. And Adam loved her for it.

So, apparently, did Charlotte.

'I'm not sad any more, Daddy,' she said. 'I'm happy.'

'I'm glad you're happy, button.'

'I'm happy because I love Dr Sam and she's okay.'

Adam could see the way his daughter's face was glowing in the dim, faintly pink light from the mushroom. She *was* happy. Totally living in the moment, her earlier upset forgotten. And she was sleepy again. She snuggled down beneath her duvet, unable to keep her eyes open any longer.

How could he cast a shadow on that happiness by suggesting that the future might hold something dark? Maybe Charlie was right and it would never happen?

And, even if it did, was the possibility of that sadness enough to overshadow the joy that could be experienced before then?

Adam ducked his head to plant a soft kiss on Charlotte's cheek.

'Night night, darling,' he whispered. 'Love you.'

He walked slowly towards the kitchen.

'Life's quite simple, really, isn't it?' he said to his mother. 'You just need to look at it through the eyes of a five-year-old.'

'Oh? All sorted, then?'

'I guess. Charlie's happy. She's asleep.'

The glance he received was soft. 'How 'bout you? Are you happy?'

She covered the slight hesitation on his part by gesturing towards the stove instead. It looked as if a pot of her famous vegetable soup was simmering and there was some fresh bread sliced on a board in front of the toaster. 'You hungry?'

Adam was still considering his answer to her question and he'd just realised he couldn't answer it just yet.

'You go ahead without me. I need to pop out again for a bit. If you're happy to stay?'

'You do whatever you need to do, love,' Jude said. 'I'm as happy as a clam.'

Adam gave her a quick kiss and then headed for his front door yet again.

Yeah…there was something he *really* needed to do.

CHAPTER THIRTEEN

THE SOONER SHE LEFT, the better.

That Adam had said so himself had broken her heart.

Sam's last day at Coromandel Hospital was supposed to be next week but she had some annual leave she hadn't taken and if a new locum hadn't arrived before then it was quite likely that either Jake or Isla would be happy to cover a shift or two for her.

It wasn't as if she had much to pack. Sam had avoided collecting things like furniture or knick-knacks in the same way she had avoided taking responsibility for a pet or a pot plant. The same way she'd been so careful not to get attached to people or places that might make it difficult to keep moving on. Right now, it felt as if she'd taken a wrong direction somewhere along the line. She'd ended up with an amazing career but not that much of a life.

She could pack up all her possessions and get them into the back of her vehicle to travel to Wellington, but this time it wasn't going to be easy or exciting to make a fresh start. It felt, in fact, as if it was going to be the hardest thing Sam had ever done in her life.

Having splashed cold water on her face to rinse off any evidence of the first tears that had escaped her eyes since the night Robbie had died, Sam put the kettle on to make a pot of tea. While it boiled, she found a notepad and pen and started scribbling a list of everything she needed to do before she left this apartment, like paying her rent until the end of the month, arranging for a final power reading and disconnecting her Wi-Fi.

She took a mug off one of the hooks on the wall and then went to the fridge to get some milk. As always, her gaze was caught by the picture held onto the door with small round magnet buttons. The picture Charlotte Carter had drawn of her, in a red cape like the superhero the little girl believed she was.

Superheroes never had families, did they?

Did they ever get *this* lonely?

The wobbly writing underneath the picture was a little blurry.

I hugged the Kauri tree. I hugged Dr Sam too. Charlie XXX

Sam's breath came out in a long, slow sigh. She took the picture off the fridge, folding it carefully as she put it on the table. She was going to tuck it away with the few other items that were precious enough to keep forever. The electric kettle flicked off, but a very different sound broke the silence that followed almost instantly.

A knock at her front door.

Not the sharp rap of an angry man. This knock was almost tentative, but Sam still knew who was going to be standing there when she opened the door.

And there he was. Tall, rumpled and obviously tired, but just as gorgeous as he had been the first time Sam had laid eyes on this man and wondered if he was a celebrity like a movie star. Despite holding his gaze without even blinking, she couldn't quite interpret his expression. Her first instinct was that it was hopeful, but why on earth would it be?

There was certainly a hint of sadness there. Because she was leaving? Because this was going to be as difficult for him as it was for her, but neither of them had any choice because of the futures that were already so firmly mapped out for each of them.

Perhaps it was apologetic? Because they were losing something special. Or maybe he had decided that his anger for her upsetting Charlotte had been misplaced.

Or maybe he'd just come back so that he could say a private goodbye?

Sam still hadn't broken the eye contact. She was trying to convey that if that was why he was here, it was a bad idea.

A very bad idea.

She knew exactly how it would end up if they found time for a private conversation and the thought of having sex with Adam knowing it had to be the last time ever was unbearable.

Because it wouldn't simply be having sex, would it?

It would be making love, as far as she was concerned, anyway. With every moment something delicious and exquisite and meaningful.

And totally impossible?

Yeah…

'I don't do relationships… But I definitely do kids…'

Even if Adam felt anything like the same way as she did, Sam knew he would sacrifice what he desired in order to keep Charlotte safe. She could imagine feeling the same way if Charlotte was *her* daughter.

Her thoughts flashed past with the astonishing speed

they were capable of, but it was still a noticeably long time to be staring at someone.

Adam's eyebrow twitched. 'Can I come in?' he asked. 'I just want to talk to you. I'm not angry. Not now…'

Sam stepped back to allow him to come inside. She pushed the front door closed, trying very hard not to remember that they'd actually had sex for the first time against this very door, while their fish and chips had been getting stone cold on the hall table.

Oh, man…

Sam had to clear her throat. 'Would you like a cup of tea? I've just boiled the kettle.'

Adam blinked at the polite query, as well he might. It was his lips that twitched this time. Hiding a smile?

'Thank you. I'd like that.'

He sat down at the table as she collected another mug and put tea in the pot to brew.

She turned to find that he'd unfolded Charlotte's picture and smoothed it open. Right beside the notepad with her scribbles on it, but it was her he was looking at.

'I wanted to apologise,' he said.

Sam gave her head a tiny shake. 'You don't need to,' she said. 'I understand why you were angry. I'm the one who should be apologising. For Charlotte getting traumatised like that. I should know better than to cross professional boundaries. I *do* know better.'

'It wasn't just Charlotte being upset,' Adam said slowly. 'I was angry at myself.'

Sam abandoned the tea making. She sank slowly onto the other chair at the small table. 'Why?'

'I got a hell of a fright when you almost got hit with that rock. When I saw you hitting the side of that cliff.'

Sam licked suddenly dry lips. 'I got a bit of a fright myself.'

Adam didn't seem to have heard her. 'I thought I was about to go through losing someone again,' he said softly. 'Someone that I love. Very much…'

Sam's breath caught in her chest.

'I never wanted to go through that again,' he continued. 'And I really didn't want Charlie to have to go through it—*ever*. So I was angry that it was kind of happening anyway.'

Sam nodded. She got it. She hadn't intended falling in love with Adam either.

'I'm sorry I took it out on you,' Adam added. 'I'm sorry I said that the sooner you left, the better it would be. It's not true. It will never be true.'

Her brain pushed a rewind button.

Someone that I love. Very much… He'd been talking about *her*, hadn't he?

'Charlie's perfectly happy now,' Adam told her. 'Because you're okay—apart from your ouchie—and she loves you very much, too. She told me tonight that if she could choose anybody in the world to be her mummy, it would be you.'

A sound broke through Sam's lips. A sound of pain.

Adam heard that. He reached out and covered her hands with his but he didn't stop talking. 'She wanted to know, if I loved you and she loved you, why you couldn't be her mummy.'

Sam could feel the tears filling her eyes now and her voice was choked. 'What did you say?'

His voice was only a whisper. 'That maybe you didn't feel the same way.' She could hear how ragged the breath he pulled in was. 'She asked me how I knew and I said I didn't, so she suggested that I asked you. Tomorrow.' A corner of his mouth lifted. 'Only I couldn't wait till tomorrow because time's running out.' He glanced down at the notepad. 'Are you running away, Sam?'

'I thought I had to,' Sam said softly. 'To keep you safe. To keep Charlie safe.'

'It's a funny thing, safety,' Adam said. 'You can mostly keep yourself safe physically by avoiding the really wild stuff, and you can keep yourself safe emotionally by avoiding getting involved but…that's not what life's about, is it? If you end up completely safe, your life ends up being pretty empty, doesn't it? We all need people. We all need family.'

Sam had dropped her gaze. She was staring at their hands. 'I don't deserve a family,' she whispered. 'I couldn't keep my best friend safe and he was the only real family I ever had. How could I be trusted with a child? Or…or a baby?'

Adam's grip tightened on her hands. 'You can't make other people's choices for them, Sam. You can only make your own. And…accidents happen. Yeah, they happen more often if you're doing something really dangerous but they can happen anyway and…if you try too hard to avoid them, you might miss out on the best stuff that there is in life. Like families.' He picked up her hand and pressed his lips to it. 'And love…'

'I do love you,' Sam said. 'But you said it yourself. It could never work. I'm too wild.'

'You are who you are,' Adam countered. 'And you're amazing. Exciting. Perfect. I love everything about you. I can learn to live with the risk and make the most of every moment we get together, but there are bigger problems, aren't there? Your dream job will never be here. We don't even have a helicopter service.'

'We have an emergency department. And a search and rescue organisation. Seems like I've had more than enough excitement in my job since I've been here.' It was true. Sam had been running towards what she had thought was her dream. A career. Now she knew that the real dream was what she had been running away from. The attachment to people. And places. From permanence and commitment and…love…

That was never going to happen now. Even if Adam was frowning at her as if he could read her thoughts and didn't believe them.

'Maybe I'm the real problem,' he said. '*I'm* too boring.'

'Are you kidding?' Sam could feel a smile starting to emerge from somewhere deep inside her. From her heart? 'You're a rock, Adam Carter. You're everything I could ever want, but you're not boring.'

The smile was reaching her lips now.

'Boring people don't put their hand up to fly off to the top of a mountain to look for someone who might be hurt,' she continued. 'And they don't make the best dad a little girl could ever, ever have.' She caught her breath. 'And they certainly don't have front door sex while their fish and chips get cold.' Her smile had widened but now it wobbled. 'I love you, Adam Carter. And I love Charlie.'

'So if we really, really want you to stay and become a part of our family, would you think about it?'

Sam shook her head, but then realised that Adam was misinterpreting it.

'I don't need to think about it,' she said in a rush. 'Of

course I'll stay. I can't imagine wanting to be anywhere else. Or *with* anyone else. I love you *so* much.'

'I love you more.'

Somehow, they were both on their feet, hugging each other so tightly it was impossible to breathe, but then Adam loosened the hold enough to let him kiss her.

Slowly.

Thoroughly.

And then he drew back just far enough to speak, but still so close that Sam could feel the movement of his lips.

'So I can tell Charlie you might be okay with the idea of being part of our family? You do realise you might need to wear a matching superhero outfit sometimes?'

'Only if you wear one, too,' she murmured. 'You're the one being brave here, Adam. Taking the risk—for you *and* Charlie.'

'No.' Adam was about to kiss her again. 'The real risk would be in letting you go.'

EPILOGUE

Five years later...

IT WAS A perfect day for a forest walk. The sun filtered through the canopy of tall trees and the huge punga ferns provided some welcome shade on a summer's afternoon.

The sound of native bird calls mingled with the calls and laughter of children, but this wasn't a school trip.

This was an outing for a group of close friends—two families that were made up of four adults and a bunch of kids that ranged in age from two years to fifteen.

'Why couldn't Ben come?' Charlotte asked.

'Because this forest has kiwis in it,' Arlo told her. 'And dogs can kill kiwis.'

'Ben wouldn't hurt a fly,' Charlotte pronounced.

'He's getting too old to walk up a big hill like this anyway.' Arlo sounded sad enough for his parents, Jake and Isla, to exchange a glance.

Adam and Sam also shared a moment of silent communication.

'Have you told him yet?' Sam asked.

'No.' Jake paused to put three-year-old Tayla down on the track now that they were over a patch of rough tree roots.

Tayla's twin brother, Harley, was trying to catch up with Arlo and Charlotte.

'We didn't want to distract him,' Isla added. 'Not when he had the junior surf competition coming up. It's bad enough to have the twins as two little shadows. If they all knew about the new puppy that's coming, the excitement level would have been through the roof and he wouldn't have got a moment's peace and quiet.' She turned to Sam. 'Are you ready for what's coming your way? I can't believe you guys decided to get one of the litter as well.'

'Charlie's been begging for a dog for years,' Adam said. 'And these ones are Ben's great-great-grand-puppies. How could we pass on that?'

'And Georgie's old enough to know not to poke its eyes,' Sam added. She grinned at her daughter, who was riding in a pack on her father's back.

'Daddy's ears aren't handles,' she said. 'Can you let them go?'

'No.' It was Georgina's favourite new word, always delivered with a wide smile.

'I don't mind,' Adam said. Remarkably, he was smiling too.

It was a slow walk uphill, to let the small children go at their own pace and enjoy their environment.

'That's a punga fern,' Arlo told Harley. 'Look…it's silver under the green side. That's why they're called silver ferns sometimes.'

Harley was watching a pair of small black and white birds darting close to the humans and making squeaking sounds like tiny kisses. He pointed up with a huge grin. 'Fern tails!' he announced triumphantly.

'Fantails,' Charlotte corrected. 'Tayla? Do you want to hold my hand to come up the steps?'

Harley was already scrambling up the steps. 'Keep an

eye on him, Arlo,' Jake called. 'The stream and the bridge are just around the next corner.'

Arlo lengthened his stride. 'I'm on it.'

The suspension bridge that had been washed away in the flood had been repaired and strengthened long ago, but this was the first time Sam and Adam had been back on this track since the first day they'd met.

They both stopped, holding hands as they watched Charlotte confidently crossing the bridge. Jake scooped up Tayla and Arlo was giving Harley a piggyback with Isla right behind them.

'Look a bit different to the last time we were here,' Adam said.

'It does,' Sam agreed.

'A bit boring?'

Sam looked at the picture-perfect stream gurgling over its rocky bed with the lush native forest on either side.

'Not boring at all,' she said. 'I had enough excitement to last a lifetime before I met you. I don't mind if it comes along every now and then, but I'm not ever going to go hunting for it again.'

She didn't need to. She had a job she loved, good friends who were also her colleagues, a community she was proud to be a part of and a family she'd never dreamed she would be lucky enough to call her own.

And it had all started right here. A long time ago now. Long enough for Sam to know she could trust everything about it. Especially her husband—the love of her life.

'That's where Miss Kempsey broke her ankle,' Charlotte was telling Arlo as they reached the other side of the bridge. 'And it was Mummy who came to save her.'

That made Adam smile. 'When was it that you stopped being Dr Sam?'

'About the same time I became Mrs Carter. Or was it when that Supergirl outfit finally fell apart?'

'You never did get your own costume. Sorry 'bout that.'

'I'm not.' Sam laughed. 'I'm not sure that it would be appreciated in Coromandel Hospital's ED department and it would definitely not be appropriate on a Land-SAR callout.'

'Come on, you two,' Isla shouted. 'We're going to see the Kauri tree.'

They all wandered uphill a little further until they came to one of the iconic trees of the New Zealand native forest. The smooth grey bark of this ancient tree was decorated with lichen and stretched up in a straight column far enough for them to have to tip their heads back to see the horizontal branches high above them.

'We were going to take a photograph for the school newsletter that day,' Charlotte reminded Adam. 'We were all going to hold hands and see how many people it took to go right round the trunk but it never happened.'

'Want to do it now?' Adam asked. 'I reckon we've got about enough people if the little guys help.'

'Ooh…yes…' Charlotte said. 'Can we?'

Of course they could. Adam took off his pack but it was Charlotte who lifted her little sister out.

'Come on, Georgie. Let's go and hug the tree.'

They made a circle around the trunk. With a lot of laughter, they managed to get the twins holding hands with Arlo between them and Jake and Isla on either side. Sam held Charlotte's hand on one side and Georgie's on the other. Jake slipped out of the circle after Adam was in place because they had plenty of people to hug the tree and he wanted to get a photo.

'I'd better be quick,' he muttered. 'The twins will get bored and take off any second.'

Adam caught Sam's gaze as he stretched out his hand to grab hers when Georgie let it go so that she could hang onto her mother's legs.

'What about you?' he murmured. 'You're not about to get bored and take off, are you?'

'You can stop asking that,' Sam said, smiling right into his eyes. 'You know I have everything I could ever want. Our life is perfect.'

'It is.' Adam was still holding her gaze. 'But I'll never ever get tired of hearing you tell me.'

'That's okay,' Sam told him. 'I'll never ever get tired of telling you.'

* * * * *

*If you missed the previous story in
the Coastside ER duet, then check out*

A Family Made in the ER

*And if you enjoyed this story, check out these other
great reads from Alison Roberts*

Single Dad's Christmas Wish
Their Fake Date Rescue
Midwife's Three-Date Rule

All available now!

MILLS & BOON®

Coming next month

THE PARAMEDIC ROOMMATE PACT
JC Harroway

'Sometimes life doesn't make much sense,' he said, his gaze lingering on her mouth for a few exhilarating seconds during which Kaia became increasingly convinced that he wanted her too.

'It makes no sense to me that a guy would walk away from you.'

A thrilling gasp sounded in her head. 'You're just saying that because you're my friend,' she pointed out, almost from habit, clinging to her last shred of willpower.

Their jokes often bordered on flirtation. But Levi's expression wasn't friendly. It was intense and searing and raging with need.

'I *am* your friend,' he confirmed, the look on his face and the few cryptic words he'd spoken, flooding her pelvis with liquid heat that slid down her legs so she feared she might actually collapse.

Drunk on the excitement pounding through her body but safe in the knowledge that he cared about her, that she trusted him, she slowly raised her hands to his shoulders.

'Well on that note, happy birthday,' she whispered.

She rose onto the tips of her toes and pressed her lips to his. Brief. Forbidden. And so tempting she couldn't breathe.

Continue reading

THE PARAMEDIC ROOMMATE PACT
JC Harroway

Available next month
millsandboon.co.uk

COMING SOON!

We really hope you enjoyed reading this book.
If you're looking for more romance
be sure to head to the shops when
new books are available on

Thursday 26th February

To see which titles are coming soon, please visit
millsandboon.co.uk/nextmonth

MILLS & BOON

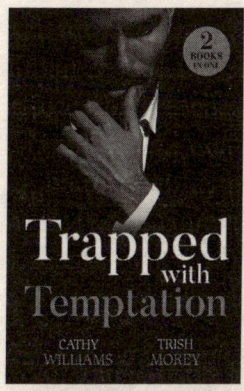
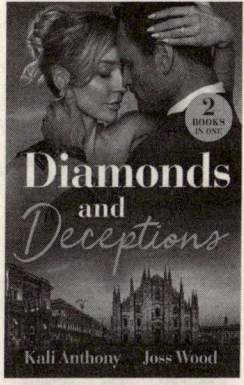
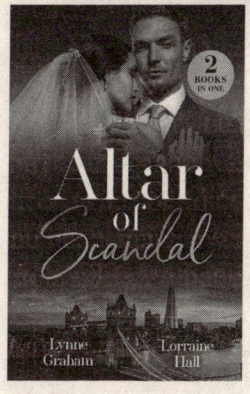
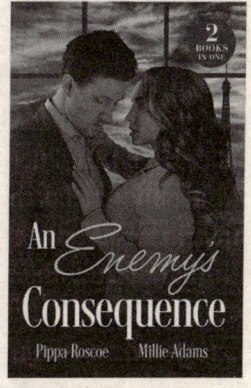

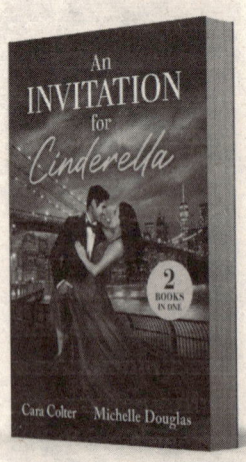
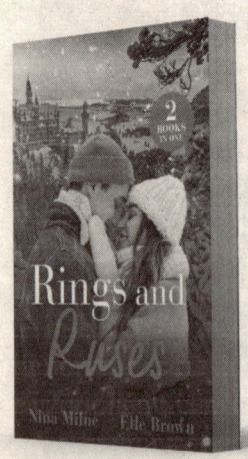

OUT NOW!

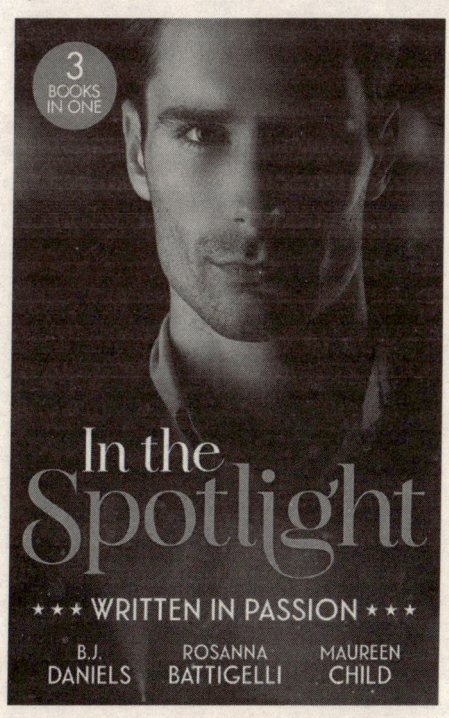

3 BOOKS IN ONE

In the
Spotlight

★★★ WRITTEN IN PASSION ★★★

B.J. DANIELS   ROSANNA BATTIGELLI   MAUREEN CHILD

Available at
millsandboon.co.uk

MILLS & BOON

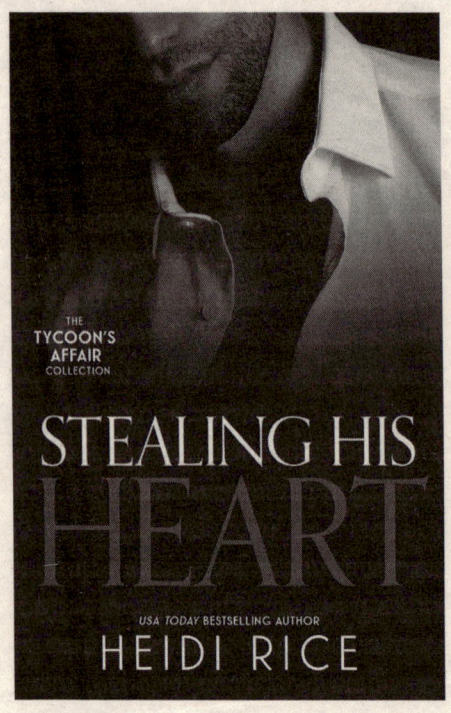

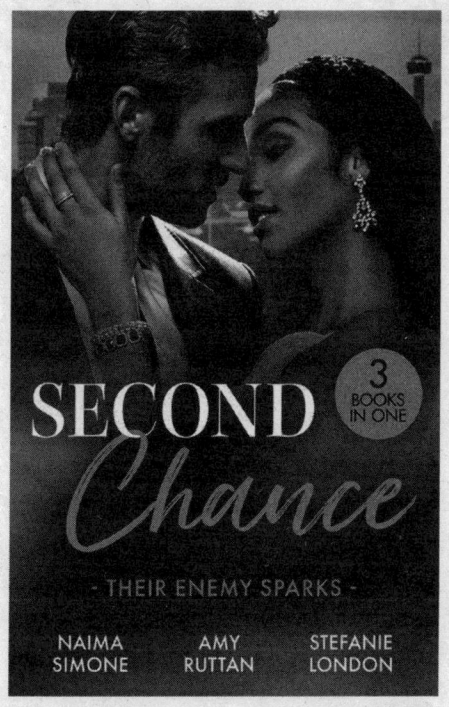